"I fart in your general di

"I fart in your general direction!"
Flatulence in Popular Culture

DON H. CORRIGAN

McFarland & Company, Inc., Publishers
Jefferson, North Carolina

ISBN (print) 978-1-4766-9196-1
ISBN (ebook) 978-1-4766-5028-9

Library of Congress and British Library
Cataloguing data are available

Library of Congress Control Number 2023028594

Front cover images © 2023 Adobe Stock/CSA-Archive

Printed in the United States of America

*McFarland & Company, Inc., Publishers
Box 611, Jefferson, North Carolina 28640
www.mcfarlandpub.com*

To the unsung heroes of our internal plumbing.
Gastrointestinal doctors deserve our gratitude
for keeping the gas works fully operational.

Also worthy of recognition are the hundreds of thousands
of fraternity brothers who have removed flatulence
from the back burner—for demonstration, discussion,
and imaginative description.

Contents

Acknowledgments

Many scholars, researchers, journalists and university colleagues as well as friends and family merit acknowledgment for inspiring and contributing to this book. As mentioned in the book's dedication, I feel particular indebtedness to doctors of gastroenterology, named and unnamed, who provided invaluable counsel on flatulence as a medical issue. Some physicians in the field are compelled to air their grievances with the journalism community. The physicians contend there is a paucity of serious exposition on flatulence that could serve the general public.

Dr. John Eckrich and Dr. Charles J. Sigmund of St. Louis were the sources for my first published words on the travails of bloating and unintended gas passing. In my initial interviews with these doctors some thirty years ago, I was fascinated to learn about the three major causes of human flatulence. That fascination has continued unabated, as evidenced by Chapter 4 in this book. The chapter details the dietary and motility factors behind flatulence as well as the persistent flatus problems for the air swallowers among us.

After my initial article on holiday flatulence quoting the doctors, I was rewarded with two tokens of appreciation for taking on a topic that is generally shunned. The first gift came from my Missouri representative in the state legislature, Francis "Bud" Barnes, who gave me a copy of his book on the great French "fartiste," Le Pétomane. I have kept this intriguing biography close at hand. My heart sometimes burns for it. I have consulted the story of Le Pétomane often over the years and am elated that I am finally able to put it to use in this treatise.

The second gift that came out of the blue after my 1992 flatulence article was a very large box, delivered on the doorstep, containing a lifetime supply of Beano. Perhaps it's appropriate at this juncture to acknowledge the inventor of Beano, a medication intended to quiet the noise and quell the fumes resulting from excessive farting after high-fiber meals. Beano was developed in 1990 by Alan Kligerman of AkPharma after more than a decade of company research into gas-causing vegetables. I think those who have benefited from Beano would surely observe a moment of silence to honor the work of this genius, Alan Kligerman.

In the three decades before my encounter with the work of Mr. Kligerman, I was companion to a diverse mix of males fixated on flatulence at the grade school, high school, college, and later the university graduate school level of education. From boys to men, they all deserve notice and gratitude for many hours of flatulence demonstrations and discussions. If there is one section of this book in which their contributions are readily apparent, it is the third chapter, "Farts Classified: Spiders, Ducks, and Squeakers." I am certain that this chapter captures only a fraction of the vast "folk vocabulary" of flatulence imparted over the years by fine fellows and friends.

One always wonders as one approaches the twilight years just how valuable one's college and university training have been—when sizing up accomplishments of a lifetime. This volume helps make such an assessment a rather facile task for me. At Knox College in Illinois, my English professors, including Dr. Howard Wilson, Dr. William Brady, Robin Metz, and Dr. Robert Hellenga, introduced me to flatulence episodes in the great works of Chaucer, Fielding, Swift, and several American authors of note. Their instruction could be described as setting the foundation for any astute observations in Chapter 5 on farts in Anglo-American literature.

At the graduate school level, I cannot help but single out my discussions and collaborations with Dr. Ralph Lowenstein and Dr. John C. Merrill at the University of Missouri Graduate School of Journalism. Merrill introduced me to his analysis of world philosophers and their impact on journalism concepts and practices. It was a short step from there for me to take their philosophies on free expression in journalism, as articulated by Merrill, and apply them to free expression in the realm of flatulence. This application manifests itself in Chapter 14, "Waxing Philosophically About Farts." Merrill's ideas were indispensable in this effort. The ideas can be found in his unique and enlightening study *Legacy of Wisdom*.

This author has been extremely fortunate to have pursued two careers simultaneously: one as a newspaper editor and the other as a college professor. The newspaper position permitted me to experiment with reader content and to assess the results. Reader reactions to my publishing articles on flatulence were immediate and unequivocal. I am grateful to these readers and must concede that the vitality of their responses was a major factor in why I took on the mission of writing this book.

In my career as a college professor of journalism and mass communications, I have experienced the intellectual stimulation of joining and participating in a number of professional organizations. Those organizations range from College Media Advisers to Associated Collegiate Press to the

Association for Education in Journalism and Mass Communications. The organization I wish to acknowledge for the purposes of this book is the Popular Culture Association, which encourages research and writing on a wide range of esoteric topics.

I have been a member of the Popular Culture Association for more than a score of years, and my work has been primarily with the Men's Studies Division which researches masculine identities and male and female gender issues. I am most indebted to professors who have headed this division and encouraged my research, including Dr. Merry Perry of West Chester University of Pennsylvania and Dr. James Alan Temple of St. Mary's College of California. My research with the Men's Studies Division of the Popular Culture Association was useful in constructing several chapters in this book, including Chapter 11, "Farts: All About Male Bonding," and Chapter 12, "Farting Goddesses Air Grievances."

The Popular Culture Association has served as a venue for introduction to a number of valuable institutions both nationally and internationally, including the American Writers Museum in Chicago, the McLuhan Institute in San Francisco, the McLuhan Centre for Culture and Technology in Toronto, the Museum of Pop Culture in Seattle, and the National Comedy Museum of Jamestown, New York. The comedy museum in particular was an important source for information on stand-up comedians and comedy trailblazers such as George Carlin. The comedy museum also offered advice on obtaining images for this book.

Two institutions not affiliated in any way with the Popular Culture Association, but which nonetheless had an impact on this book, are the Creation Museum and the Ark Encounter in Kentucky. Both of these museums provided some of the inspiration for Chapter 2, "Fanning the Flames of Fart Conspiracies." The amazing Creation Museum offers a colorful, if questionable, explanation of the origin of the universe, based on a literal interpretation of the Genesis creation narrative in the Bible. Similarly, the Ark Encounter, based on the Genesis flood story contained in the Bible, provided some content for this book in regard to biblical tales and flatulence in the Old Testament.

As an academic, I have witnessed many campus demonstrations over the years. As a newspaper journalist, I have covered labor marches, anti-war demonstrations, protests by men's rights groups and by women's right activists, and other actions involving civil rights. Protest tactics always are a part of these stories, but in my years of covering these events, I was never introduced to the infamous "fart-ins" devised by the much-maligned protest tactician Saul Alinsky.

Nevertheless, upon learning of Alinsky's enthusiasm for "fart-in" actions used by his activist acolytes, there was no question that a description of flatulence protest methodology belonged in this book. These accounts appear in Chapter 13, "Protest Farts: We Shall Not Be Moved." My interest in the postulations of protest tacticians can be credited to past acquaintances such as Michael Cavanaugh of the U.S. labor movement, Mary Daly of the women's movement, and David Usher of the fathers' rights and men's movement.

Finally, the assistance and patience of my family should be acknowledged here. My wife, Susanne, exhibited exemplary endurance and forbearance as I viewed far too many films with flatulence episodes. Especially annoying for her were the Mike Myers Austin Powers films with such characters as Alotta Fagina and Fat Bastard. The children's fart films proved equally annoying with flatulence making its presence known in such popular tyke fare as *The Lion King* and *George of the Jungle.* Nevertheless, Susanne knew that all of this malodorous movie viewing was necessary for my comprehensive Chapter 9, "Farts in Film: Memorable Masterpieces."

My own children, Brandon and Christa, also have provided valuable assistance with this book. At an early age, they took a deep dive into the Grossology series of books in the kids' sections of the local Barnes & Noble and Borders bookstores. Their enthusiasm for gross content paved the way for my acceptance of the subsequent line of children's fart books, covered here in Chapter 6, "Noise Over Children's Fart Books." As youngsters, my thoughtful children were always there for dear old dad with fart gag gifts on birthdays and Father's Days and at Christmas. These most memorable occasions, with their wonderful expressions of love, were the genesis for Chapter 10, "Merchandising of Fart Gifts."

Special kudos should be accorded to the editorial staff of the newspaper I have been associated with for four decades, the weekly *Webster-Kirkwood Times* in St. Louis. My news colleagues, Jaime Mowers and Melissa Wilkinson, were most supportive with quirky flatulence anecdotes, sometimes involving their own relatives. Ursula Ruhl and Kevin Murphy were extremely helpful in offering their unique skills and advice on images for the book. Flatulence is not photogenic. Gas is gossamer. Farts are diaphanous. Images for this book presented a challenge.

More special kudos have to go out to the folks at the crown prince of popular culture books, McFarland, in Jefferson, North Carolina. Managing Editor Layla Milholen always has been receptive to my offbeat book ideas, whether they involve red squirrels and Marshall McLuhan, roadkill jewelry and recipes for fresh roadkill possum, or flatulence in mass media and popular culture.

Book writing can be a grind. I especially appreciated the kind note from McFarland President Rhonda Herman after I signed on for this project:

"Don, this is our third collaboration. You pick fun topics and are delightful to work with. Thanks for adding smiles to the McFarland catalog and our work lives." Well, thank you, Rhonda, for the vote of confidence. I am so pleased to be able to deliver the goods—a virtual flatulence potpourri—and on deadline.

Introduction

Clearing the Air: Fart Disinformation

Many millennia ago, there were farts. Hundreds of millions of years ago, below the surface of the oceans, single-celled microbes were passing methane gas. Aquatic creatures followed. Long before the fish developed appendages and crawled out of the oceans to evolve into land-based creatures, the fish were passing gas. Dinosaurs and other giant reptiles came onto the scene and were releasing their own flatulence, and in high volume. The small mammals who hid in fear of the dinosaurs some 200 million years ago—and who were our ancestors—also were passing gas.

Farts happen—and they happened. They happened without the presence of human beings, but when humans came along, they instinctively took ownership of them. Too bad for lowly farts, because humans insisted on making farts a part of their extravagant and convoluted storytelling. Cavemen farted around primeval campfires and soon told boisterous tales about their farts. Flatulence became a part of the oral culture of mankind. This persisted for thousands of years, until the mechanical age and the electronic age of man changed everything.

An oral culture transformed into a mechanical culture, which was quickly overwhelmed by an electronic culture. The mechanical age brought the printing press and newspaper accounts in black and white about farting. The electronic age followed. At first, the electronics brought audio accounts of farting distributed over radio waves. However, human tales of farting were soon transmitted over television broadcasts and captured on the big screen of film houses and motion picture complexes.

Today, we live in an Anthropocene Age of human dominance of the globe. It's an epoch of true facts but also of hoaxes and conspiracies. Humans cannot resist concocting versions of reality that draw on malevolent forces and nefarious activities. Great mysteries are beyond our control and they alter our fates. The examples are endless. Alien beings landed in spaceships in Roswell, New Mexico, and are still among us. Jet aircraft

1

leave contrails that are full of chemicals that are used to experiment on the populations below.

Political conspiracies frighten some, enrage others. A John Birch Society fantasy perpetuates the belief that fluoridation of water supplies will make us vulnerable to foreign enemies. Another conspiracy holds that John F. Kennedy and his son, John F. Kennedy, Jr., are cryogenically frozen in an underground bunker but will emerge when the time is right. A "deep state" cabal of globalist politicians is said to dine like cannibals and to engage in satanic, pedophiliac rituals. The pharmaceutical industry distributes vaccines that cause autism in newborns.

Now in the age of high-speed Internet and social media platforms, slow-moving parcels of misinformation accelerate into digitalized bundles of disinformation. And these packets of fraud and falsehoods have often contained outrageous fibs about flatulence. Frantic humans are left howling after the dissemination of scary fart fables in a time of pandemic. They scream: "Tear off your useless masks. They can't protect you from the virus. Deadly pathogens are being farted at you from every direction. Masks can't do anything."

Chapter 1 of this study examines the case of the so-called "Panera Karen" who shouted out an anti-mask diatribe in a California restaurant. She was convinced that the virus was escaping from nearby asses in the sandwich line. Because she believed farts were carrying the virus, she refused to protect herself or others with a mask in the pandemic. The disturbing incident revealed the destructive behavior of Americans spellbound and disabled by disinformation and, in this case, because of flatulence disinformation.

Flatulence has been a source of historic fakery, scurrilous hoaxes, fabrications, and distortions for centuries. Nevertheless, some of the outrageous stories can turn out to have an element of truth. Chapter 2 of this study examines some of the breathtaking tales and conspiracies about the impact of farts on ancient and contemporary history. Perhaps this narrative raises as many questions as it answers: Did misguided farts cause deaths and mutilations in the time of the Egyptian kings and the Roman empire? Did Adolf Hitler's chronic flatulence affect the outcome of World War II? Did attorney Rudy Giuliani's press conference defending Donald J. Trump backfire because of the incessant gas emissions from his backside?

Also examined in the second chapter on fart conspiracies is the rather peculiar omission of fart emissions in the biblical stories of Adam and Eve, David and Goliath, Jonah and the whale, and Noah and his ark. The story of Noah stretches credibility because it involves an ark at sea during 40 days of flooding of biblical proportions. Even more incredible is the proposition that this boat has two of every animal on the planet on board. The story arouses even more skepticism as we now know about the flatulence potential of all those mariners on the ark. And, yet, there is nary a mention of the hazardous air quality on a ship of many cubits but with few windows to disperse the flatulence of all the animal gas passers.

Chapter 3 of this book provides us with a vocabulary of flatulence. Any authoritative flatulence treatment must include a classification of the wide assortment of expulsions in the fart world and all their unique characteristics. English satirist and flatulence authority Jonathan Swift recognized this when he began dividing farts into categories. He offered details on several varieties of flatulence more than 250 years before this seminal work. Among the specimens of gas emissions that he described were "the sonorous and full-toned or rousing fart," "the double fart," "the soft fizzing fart," "the wet fart," and "the sullen wind-bound fart."

The third chapter in this work builds on Swift's flatulence foundation and offers the most complete fart definitions and descriptions ever assembled. Interestingly enough, many of the synonyms cited for each specimen of fart were created by the fertile minds of boys and male teens. English composition teachers must lament that the energy and creativity young males have put into constructing a virtual fart thesaurus have not expanded their vocabulary in other realms. Still, who cannot be impressed by the terminology that they have bequeathed us with such appellations as fanny floater, seam splitter, tile peeler, corn slider, trouser cough, bat skat, dog chime, goose pudding, and so many more.

Whether we're chuckling, cackling, or chortling over a corn slider or a trouser cough, the serious fact remains that millions of unhappy flatulence producers consult with their doctors annually in an attempt to get some relief. Chapter 4 takes a close look at what physicians are grappling with as they diagnose the particulars of chronic gas-passing conditions. An even tougher challenge for physicians involves a determination of the most effective prescriptions and therapies that can remedy the situations. Also of note is the progress that has been made in both the diagnosis and treatment of flatulence maladies.

Switching gears from the medical front on flatulence, Chapter 5 takes a good look at more than 500 years of gas passing in literature. The wide-ranging flatulence literary tradition in the English language began with Geoffrey Chaucer's character of Absolom climbing to the window of his love in search of a kiss, only to be met by a fart in the face. The fart tradition continues in England with William Shakespeare's plays and comedies and Henry Fielding's invention of the novel. Fielding's realism in British fiction could not ignore the very real presence of farting as part of the human condition.

When the American War of Independence succeeded against the

British colonizers and they departed, American writers began their own flatulence literary tradition. By the time of authors like J.D. Salinger and Philip Roth, American writers had blown it out of the park. Founding father Benjamin Franklin gave us a treatise on a "stinking in the breeches" that has become a benchmark for insightful essays about flatulence. In our own time, J.D. Salinger has given us classic characters like Holden Caulfield and Edgar Marsalla and the terrific farts that terrify school authorities.

Children's books constitute another genre of literature that has only recently delved into the realm of flatulence in words and images. Chapter 6 examines the "Grossness Revolution" of the 1990s in children's books, which allowed for words and images associated with gross bodily functions. It was only a matter of time before pimples, boogers, and snot gave way to what lurks below. Soon, the children's book sections of Barnes & Noble and the now-defunct Borders were filled with titles about farting faeries and unicorns, farting goldfish and canaries, farting circus clowns and restaurant cooks. By golly, everybody was farting.

Authors of children's books defended their literary efforts aimed at pint-sized readers, who all needed to know that it's simply natural for humans to pass a quart of rectal gas daily. In fact, it's not just humans who are ripping them off through the old bottom bassoon. Flatulating celebrities include the Easter Bunny, Rudolph the Red-Nosed Reindeer, and the jolly fat man himself, Santa Claus. Some moralists were critical and opined that we would reap the whirlwind for tolerating all this farting content for the young ones. But the kids loved it and soon had stories about farting leprechauns, farting penguins, farting pandas, and farting flamingos on their bookshelves and readily available for their bedtime reading.

Meanwhile, adults also were reading more and more about flatulence in their daily newspapers. Mainstream conservative newspapers took aim in editorials about the permissive atmosphere ushered in by the Grossology movement for kids. Where would it all end? Tabloid newspapers got on the bandwagon with their own brand of flatulence content. In typical, sensational, tabloid fashion, these newspapers wrote about politicians accidentally slipping out a fanny floater at a press conference. Or they wrote about bandits whose cover was blown when they farted too loudly and the cops caught wind of their hiding places.

Serious newspapers wrote legal analysis pieces on their business pages about the changing regulatory climate for broadcasters when it comes to obscenity, profanity, indecency and flatulence. The robe-attired members of the U.S. Supreme Court, as well as the judiciary at the lower court level, were making decisions in the area of "law and odor"—the subject matter for Chapter 7 of this book. Radio shock jocks and comedians like Howard

Stern needed to stop talking about privates and flatulence on broadcast stations on the old AM / FM radio frequencies or face heavy fines. However, the courts gave the all-clear for the most outrageous fart fare to air on satellite radio, cable television and subscription services. Stern moved to satellite radio.

Cable television has provided the perfect media venue for stand-up comedians intent on indulging in edgy flatulence humor. Chapter 8 provides some early examples of fart routines on cable television's Home Box Office by comedians George Carlin and Eddie Murphy. Carlin is famous for his vocal fart imitations, which he used frequently in his presentations to show his disgust with phonies and shams. Murphy will be forever remembered for his lengthy recollection of the "fart game" in the bathtub with his older brother. Fans also will forever recall his glowing orange suit on stage while delivering details about the "big brown shark" launched by his brother.

Although fart jokes and flatulence performances have traditionally been considered the sole intellectual property of male stand-up comedians, female humorists have now horned in on that same territory. This has turned out to be a gas. Among the claimants are Ali Wong, Patti Harrison, Nikki Glaser, Hayley Georgia Morris, Jade Catta-Preta, and Michelle Wolf. Nothing is off limits for some of the younger female comics. They have spent some time in Dutch ovens and are ready to talk about the clam bake experience. They can brag about their own offensive "lady farts." They will not flinch in airing out their grievances with men who don't really appreciate flatulence equity.

Cable television and satellite radio have hosted hours and hours of fart material. It's more than a little astonishing, if not mind-numbing, to think that mankind has placed satellites in orbit above Earth so that its transponders can beam down vulgar fart jokes to millions of fart aficionados. High technology in the service of delivering flatulence humor to Earth must give us pause. So too must the employment of digital audio delivery and innovative screen technology for today's cinemas to wow us with movie fart scenes.

Flatulence content in the movies is the subject matter for Chapter 9, which takes great pains to survey fart production in a host of movie productions. Unfortunately, some fart film gem is always going to be left out. Among some of the serious omissions in this chapter on movies is the famous false alarm fart scene in the Chevy Chase classic *Christmas Vacation*. When Aunt Bethany comes to the home of the Griswold family for Christmas, the old woman is gently chided for bringing unnecessary presents: "You shouldn't have done that," Ellen Griswold tells her.

Aunt Bethany, however, cannot hear well and begins apologizing:

"Oh, dear, did I break wind?" Her husband corrects her and retorts that if she had broken wind, the entire room would have cleared out. Aunt Bethany's famous holiday line is now emblazoned on T-shirts that sell like sugar cookies every year around Christmas time. Although *Christmas Vacation* is a grave omission among the fart emission movies included in Chapter 9, plenty of other cinematic offerings are presented for review.

The fart movie chapter does not attempt to rate the Top 20 or Top 50 fart scenes in the cinema. Instead movies are categorized by type for a more accessible consideration of the range of fart movies available. Categories include blue flame movies in which farts are ignited; fart bubble movies in which flatulence travels through water for dispersal; fart bully movies in which flatulence is used to embarrass or humiliate others; and flatulence in kids' movies such as the many Disney offerings.

Movies with flatulence scenes do not merely entertain us, but these cinema offerings also provide history lessons of great import. One of these lessons comes courtesy of *Monty Python and the Holy Grail*, which gives history buffs new insights into the travails of King Arthur and His Knights of the Round Table. The legend of the 13th century concerns a royal search for the holy grail and the meaning of life. When King Arthur, situated below a castle's walls with his knights, looks up and begins to question the hostile French watchman, the response is quite disconcerting: "You don't frighten us, English pig-dogs! Go and boil your bottoms.... I don't want to talk to you no more, you empty-headed animal food trough wiper! I fart in your general direction!" No more wondering about the origin of the historic strained relations between the French and English after this sordid exchange.

Flatulence may be childish at times, but flatulence is not just for kids. This becomes apparent in Chapter 10's discussion of the cornucopia of fart merchandise available for holidays, birthdays, anniversaries and more. There are fart music machines, fart pajamas, fart shorts and fart shirts, fart coffee mugs, fart warning buttons, fart hats, fart undergarments, fart pillows and cushions, fart dolls and fart teddy bears. And, of course, the Pull My Finger Farting Donald Trump Plush Doll with Animated Hair.

The next two chapters examine flatulence and gender. Chapter 11 examines the role of gas-passing in male-bonding from a very early age. In the world of nine-year-old boys, farts are the coin of the realm. A few strategic methane bombs in the school hallway or on the baseball diamond can buy a young boy a one-way ticket to "Popularityville" with his peers. Flatulence also has its place in later life for males, whether it's in the military barracks or a locker room for professional sports teams. Male flatulence behavior is all about the male-bonding.

Two things are beginning to militate against the laissez-faire farting behavior typical of men in professional sports or in the military. For one thing, women are entering the sports arena and joining the military in increasing numbers. This challenges the traditional male culture in both of these important domains. Second, the masculinist movement in America shows that men are becoming more introspective and thoughtful about what constitutes acceptable male behavior on the flatulence front.

Flatulence in the life of females is not so simple, not so easily examined. Women are in a tough spot when it comes to farting. The "goddess complex," which puts women on a pedestal, cautions against the fairer sex behaving like proudly farting men. The women who let it all hang out—and who let it waft about—can be easily dismissed as "tomboys" and mercilessly fart-shamed. Chapter 12 takes a look at the decline of the "goddess complex," but that does not mean flatulence will become normalized or feminized for women or that it will become a vehicle for female bonding.

In examining male flatulence norms, Chapter 11 analyzes eight major groups within the masculinist movement and their likely positions on flatulence expression. This task is more difficult when analyzing the women's movement because there are so many different strains of feminism to consider. Nevertheless, Chapter 11 does make an effort to delineate where feminism has taken women and American culture when it comes to flatulence. The feminist conundrum when it comes to the issue of flatulence expression will often mirror the dilemma faced by women's groups on the issue of whether pornography should or should not be protected expression. Opinions can be polarized and uncompromising.

It should come as no surprise, then, that opinions also are polarized and uncompromising on the question of whether farting is a useful form of social or political protest. Readers may be intrigued to learn about the concept of so-called "fart-in" protests in Chapter 13. Mobilization of flatulence in the service of social or political protest may be centuries old, but in our time, it has been popularized by the controversial community organizer Saul Alinsky, who died in 1972. Ironically, Hillary Clinton, an admirer of Alinsky in her college days at Wellesley, was targeted by a fart-in protest later in her political career.

There's a certain pathos and poignancy in learning about the use of farts in a student protest against guns on campus at the University of Texas at Austin. The campus is the site of one of the first mass shootings in America when in 1966 Charles Whitman climbed to the 28th floor of the clock tower with multiple guns. He shot and killed 14 people and injured 31 others. Students were no safer one-half century later when they were reduced to farting for their lives. One protester declared: "When you come to my community, to the university that I love, and you threaten the lives of my friends, what I have to say is: I'm going to fart in your face!"

Philosophers can get a little in your face with their expounding on farting. It's dumbfounding to discover how many repositories of wisdom have chosen to expend their energy on flatulence issues. Communitarians like the Chinese philosopher Confucius naturally cautioned against vulgarity and the selfishness that must include the expelling of gas in public forums. In contrast, some thinkers in the libertarian camp would be totally comfortable firing off farts with the faux cowboys seated around the campfire in the movie *Blazing Saddles*. The great essayist Michel de Montaigne counsels us not to judge too harshly those who are guilty of excessive farting.

If the noisy scene from *Blazing Saddles* seems a bit absurd, then the existential philosophers are probably worth a read with their contention that we must reckon with all the absurdities of life to arrive at truth. While the communitarians engage in debate with libertarians on the moral justification for farting in public, existentialists find the whole discussion, well, frankly, absurd. Essays on the existentialist philosophy are not just so much breaking of the wind, but some of the best expositions on existentialism actually come in the form of novels by existentialists Jean-Paul Sartre, Albert Camus, and Kurt Vonnegut. And it's Kurt Vonnegut who finally declared: "I tell you, we are here on earth to fart around, and don't let anybody tell you different."

The Postscript for this book simply provides a synopsis of some of the flatulence experiences encountered in the author's lifetime that inspired the writing of this book. It might be useful for the reader to take in this chapter before reading the rest of the book. The biographical information will shed light on how this treatise has been a pot simmering for literally decades. It's a relief to finally get these stories out there. The author invites readers to share their own flatulence life stories with their friends, relatives, and acquaintances. In these contentious times, flatulence may be the one area where we can all find community and common ground.

CHAPTER 1

Covid Conspiracy

"Not Silent, But So Deadly"

She will forever be known as "Panera Karen." She earned her unflattering nickname after she went on a tear in a Panera Bread restaurant on the West Coast. Her tirade was triggered when she was asked to put on a mask to protect herself and others from the Covid-19 virus. Her clamorous refusal to comply was not such an unusual occurrence in itself in 2020.

During the pandemic, plenty of Americans erupted in anger about the loss of their "individual liberty" when asked to wear a protective mask in the company of others. Plenty of irritable Americans expressed outrage over the health directives of public officials and restaurant managers. These "freedom fighters" resisted the medical community's directives and likened the officials and restaurant managers to despots like Hitler, Mussolini, and Stalin.

What made Panera Karen's meltdown a little different is that she mixed her obscenity-laced cries of resistance with the twisted logic of a spreading Covid-19 fart conspiracy. In the disturbance at a Panera Bread in Chico, California, Panera Karen yelled at other customers who were upset by her refusal to follow precautions and to wear a mask. She belittled their intelligence and screamed that the masks were useless; she claimed the deadly virus could be spread through wafting farts. She bolstered her high decibel explanation by declaring that since you can smell farts through the masks, it's obvious that the coverings provide no real protection. Smelling is believing—the virus microbes could hitchhike on the creeping odor of flatus, infiltrate the tightest of masks, and enter the nasal passages and beyond in search of some vital organs to degrade and destroy.

"You think that mask is going to protect you?" the woman screamed at one of her detractors in the restaurant. "You fart out your ass! You can smell it out of your ass! You think that mask is going to protect you?"[1] Who could argue with her high-pitched conviction? She fancied herself a kind of Paula Revere of the restaurant world with her warning that the red-coated balls of viral infection were coming—and they could be transported through the hot air mass of a mess of flatulence. Panera Karen did not receive plaudits for her bravery in warning others about the false security of masks in the face of filthy, floating viral fart wind. She found herself demeaned by the other customers. She was castigated by Panera employees. She was later interred and eviscerated on the Internet. She was humiliated in news headlines and on blogs.

At the time of the incident, Panera employees reassured customers that the woman would not be served and that security personnel would soon be out to deal with her situation. She would have to leave the premises. Customers took cell phone videos of the event and one cursed her for her selfishness and stupidity. Her obstreperous behavior was posted on the web and the post immediately went viral, along with the horrified reactions of web viewers watching Panera Karen in action. The *New York Post* reported on the melee and headlined the story "'Panera Karen' claims masks won't stop Covid-19 since pants don't contain farts."[2] She earned the appellation "Karen," which has been bestowed on tens of thousands of women who appear to act "entitled" and who are prone to disorderly outbursts if they are offended and do not get their way.

Panera Karen had her detractors but also more than a few allies in her battle against protective coverings. U.S. president Donald Trump mocked the wearing of masks and said they looked ridiculous. Many American governors followed the president's lead, including Missouri governor Mike Parson who derided "the dang mask" and balked at mandating its use.[3] Panera Karen received much support on the web from mask haters who declared wearers "to be the dumbest group of sheep ever seen." She was praised for her spirit of independence against "these 'men' afraid of a woman because she's not an ignorant order-follower like them." One observer applauded Panera Karen for showing the critical need for fart-proof disposable adult undergarments. This kind of underwear would be far more protective than a mask and let you "cut the cheese, tear ass and flatulate without spreading deadly viruses."[4]

Those opposing Panera Karen were particularly outraged when she puckered up and intentionally blew in the face of another restaurant customer. She huffed and puffed and blew as if to make light of others' fears of being exposed to germs and catching the virus. "Deliberately breathing on someone, especially during a pandemic, is assault. I hope the police find this woman and throw her in jail. If she has a job working for a company, then I hope they also see this video and fire her," commented one observer.

"Can't believe someone can be so disgusting and crude," wrote another. "Hope she remembers her behavior when she is on a ventilator."

Others took Panera Karen to task for actually believing and espousing the view that human farts could spread the virus. Taking aim and hurling these kinds of aspersions on the all–American fart, making flatulence the bad guy in a 100-year pandemic, seemed to be a move right out of Vladimir Putin's playbook.[5]

2020: *Year of the Panera, Pandemic, and Poots*

In 2020, America and the world came to realize that a viral pandemic could be more destructive and lethal than a devastating global war. As millions of people became infected and fatalities mounted, serious questions were raised: Why were so many people across the globe so ill prepared for this deadly disease? How did thriving economies collapse so quickly with the viral onslaught? What was the effect of so many people refusing to wear protective face coverings in this contagious pandemic? And last but not least: Could this highly volatile Covid-19 virus really be spread far and wide by a careless release of contaminated flatulence?

Panera Karen embraced one of the many conspiracy theories that always get formulated and fomented in a time of serious crisis. This theory maintained that a deadly virus could, indeed, be spread by the passing of farts. Accusatory fingers were raised and pointed in the direction of the world's buttocks. As has happened so often in the past, the much-maligned fart was again scapegoated, this time for spreading a Covid-19 virus in a serious pandemic. From the beginning of time, farting has taken the fall for all manner of human misfortune. Farts have been blamed for disastrous wars, pestilence and the rise of terrible dictators. Farts have taken it on the rim for global warming, climate change, the loss of ice at Earth's poles as well as for murderous super storms and killer wildfires. Farts have been blamed for the wipeout of entire species.

Outrageous fart conspiracies are readily accepted and repeated by all those susceptible to dubious speculation, destructive pseudo-science, or questionable folklore. Fart conspiracies appeal to those with a healthy—or an especially unhealthy—skepticism toward everything. These are folks who cannot accept the scientific explanation for what decimated the dinosaurs. It was not the fiery light and heat of a descending asteroid that incinerated the Brontosaurus and the Stegosaurus. A more likely explanation for their extinction among the conspiracy theorists has to involve dinosaur farts.

These are the same folks who attempt to understand the factors behind the rise of Nazism and the dictator Adolf Hitler and then are inclined to believe it had something to do with der Führer's irritable bowel syndrome, bloating, and backside issues. If they want to know what has been caus-ing the polar ice caps to melt and the seas to rise, they are predisposed to believe that it has less to do with any belching industrial smokestacks or car exhaust and much more to do with cattle and humans emitting methane gas around the world. Or is it maybe a combination of the two?

In the case of the global tragedy of Covid-19, farts became a prime suspect within weeks of the spread of the disease. Although the virus was thought to have originated with bats sold for human consumption in a so-called "wet market" for food in Wuhan, China,[6] the spread of the dis-ease was soon pinned on so-called "wet farts" originating from millions of posteriors on the planet. Theories on a fart-driven transmission of the virus were taken seriously and examined by medical professionals.

Newspapers, magazines, and Internet sites wasted no time draw-ing from the numerous studies of medical experts. The media then put their own spin on the experts' fart findings. Fart theories on the spread of the virus were posted on the worldwide web—and like just about everything else in 2020—the theories went viral. Peo-ple were rightly bewildered. Were these theories on fla-tus spreading coronavirus just noxious nonsense and fart fake news? Or should they be examined, and be-lieved, and re-circulated?

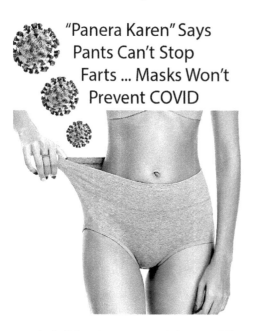

"Panera Karen" Says Pants Can't Stop Farts ... Masks Won't Prevent COVID

A California woman, nicknamed "Panera Karen" by the news media, argued that face masks are useless to stop the spread of Covid. She shouted in a Panera restaurant in July 2020 that the virus could be spread via con-taminated fart releases (graphic by Kevin Murphy).

Panera Karen certainly embraced the Covid-19 fart transmission proposition. It was not fake news for Panera Karen. She was not at all reticent about sharing this shaky piece of the puzzling pandemic story. She became a co-conspirator in dissem-inating the disinformation involving the Covid-19 fart transmission theory. She shouted it aloud in a restau-rant full of vulnerable cus-tomers quietly ordering their broccoli cheddar soup, lemon drop cookies, and bear claws.

She let them know her conviction that a mask is no defense against a pandemic when farts are aloft: "You fart out your ass! You can smell it out of your ass! You think that mask is going to protect you?" Panera Karen screamed.[7]

Real Poop on Aerosol Flatulence

Covid-19 can be transmitted through a variety of means, including the contaminated aerosol of a sneeze or a cough. The virus can also be spread through errant nasal droplets from someone who has contracted the virus. Spitting is also a foul human habit that can spread the virus. And then there is the issue of whether the virus can also be spread through a "backdoor" channel, through the voluntary and involuntary acts of farting. The Covid-19 fart transmission conspiracy theory had its origin in the discovery that the virus could be present in fecal matter, better known to the layman as poop. If tiny virus-contaminated poop particles were propelled into the air from a fart expulsion, it naturally followed that such a release could be just as harmful as a contaminated sneeze, a rasping cough, or an irresponsible secretion of spittle.

Some of the first medical discussions of the possibility of viral fart transmissions appear to have come from Down Under, specifically from Australia. In a podcast originating from the Australian Broadcasting Corporation, Dr. Norman Swan, who was hosting it, explained that farts could indeed spread the infection. Other doctors later concurred, saying that farting could be an "aerosol-generating procedure."[8] Unfortunately, the media picked up on the assertions without including all the needed qualifiers. There was no context accompanying the bald-faced proposition that farts could infect people with Covid-19 and spread the scourge like wildfire.

In the case of Dr. Swan's theorizing about infectious farts, the important qualifier was that only "bare-bottomed farting" was likely to pose a danger. Swan took pains to point out that most of us wear "masks," which cover our farts all the time. These makeshift masks include our protective garments of underwear, pants, dresses, shorts, and other clothing. Swan did caution that it's important to maintain social distancing and to not fart too close to other people and to always avoid farting with a bare bottom. A bare bottom is, indeed, capable of gas emissions containing coronavirus that could be silent but deadly.

Dr. Aaron E. Glatt, a Mount Sinai South Nassau epidemiologist and professor of medicine at the Icahn School of Medicine at Mount Sinai, issued a statement in an effort to clarify the medical community's stance on transmission of coronavirus via airborne farts: "Studies have clearly shown that a significant percentage of Covid-19 patients do have GI (gastrointestinal) symptoms (alone, or in combination with respiratory or other general symptoms) at the time of illness presentation. However, there are no published data on whether flatulence alone presents any risk of transmission, although, in a clothed person, it would be unlikely to be a significant route of transmission."[9]

The Centers for Disease Control and Prevention (CDC) also poo-pooed the Covid-19 fart transmission theory, but emphasized that infections are capable of spreading through different portals in the body such as the anus, mouth, eyes, nose, respiratory tract, broken skin, or wounds and genitals. The CDC underlined its major proviso that frequent handwashing remains one of its major recommendations for avoiding infection. Washing hands for at least 20 seconds after using the toilet also was promoted as a preferred safety practice by health professionals. Reference to toilet use inevitably brought to the fore one more precautionary measure: closing the lid before flushing the bowl. Keeping a lid on it could stop up to 80 percent of the fecal particles from being aerosolized, thus hindering the spread of the infection via a toilet plume after flushing.[10]

The lid was finally slammed down on the preposterous Covid-19 fart transmission conspiracy theory after researchers noted a scientific demonstration conducted in 2001. The turn-of-the-century study was conducted by Dr. Karl Kruszelnicki, who was dubbed by his admirers as the Bill Nye of Australia. Kruszelnicki measured and assessed the expulsions of passing gas by having a subject fart onto two Petri dishes. The farts were passed once while the subject was wearing pants and again when he was in a barebottomed state.

Kruszelnicki then described the method by which he had established whether human flatus was germ-laden or merely malodorous: "I contacted Luke Tennent, a microbiologist in Canberra, and together we devised an experiment. He asked a colleague to break wind directly onto two Petri dishes from a distance of 5 centimeters, first fully clothed, then with his trousers down. Then he observed what happened. Overnight, the second Petri dish sprouted visible lumps of two types of bacteria that are usually found only in the gut and on the skin. But the flatus which had passed through clothing caused no bacteria to sprout, which suggests that clothing acts as a filter."[11]

The 2001 results were beyond disputation and could be readily duplicated and applied to the situation with the 2020 pandemic. The conclusion was that wearing pants or other garments can block germ-laden microbes in much the same way as a mask. Skeptics might argue that the masks used in the pandemic crisis are much more porous than the clothes normally cloaking a bare bottom. Both masks and clothing are porous and not air-tight, that much is true. The question is whether the aerosol droplets carrying the microbes can penetrate and emerge from either material.

Further studies of masks and clothing material conclude that both are efficient and proven prophylactics. A mask worn properly can easily contain the viral contamination in a sneeze or a cough. Pants and undergarments can readily corral viral-infested fecal components of a fart. The possibility of dangerous droplet transmission is next to nil, according to scientists. The Covid-19 fart transmission theory was effectively nixed and blown out of the conspiratorial water.

Skeptics are still not satisfied. They might ask: So how does the smell get through pants and clothing, but the viral component remains behind? Science has the answers. Scientists point out that although farts are made of a lot of different things, it's the sulfur dioxide molecule that packs the smelly punch. The SO2 molecule consists of one sulfur atom and two oxygen atoms. That molecule is considerably smaller than the red, coronavirus sphere that the entire world now recognizes. It's a sphere with protein cylinders sticking out and it has a tough time getting through either undies or a mask.

An odoriferous SO2 molecule measures about 0.3 nanometers in diameter compared to the 100 nanometers for the diameter for the coronavirus. Therefore the ball of Covid-19 is more than 300 times larger than the sulfur dioxide that helps make a fart a fart. It should be pretty obvious how a proper mask can contain the larger coronavirus, while the tiny molecules of fart smell can go slipping right through most masks and clothing materials.[12]

Nevertheless, anti-maskers in the age of pandemic refused to acknowledge what science had to say. From their perspective, masks look silly, feel uncomfortable, steam up eyeglasses, inhibit breathing, and represent the worst of the subservient, scaredy-cat, liberal political class. And besides all that, masks are just downright ineffective, because they can't even block a simple fart, according to misguided mask opponents.

Disinformation in a Pandemic Age

When the full history of the Covid-19 pandemic's impact on the United States gets written, historians will undoubtedly express shock at the amount of disinformation that hit the country along with the spreading virus. Americans were confused and overwhelmed by distortions, exaggerations, and outright deceits disseminated on both legacy and social media. Americans had to decide what was correct information when they were repeatedly told the virus would magically disappear by the president of the United States. Donald Trump also contended that the summer heat of 2020 would end the rampaging virus, that there would be a vaccine before the November election, and that wearing masks was ineffective and should be optional at best.

It did not help that much of this information was coming from the highest places, such as the White House. It did not help that much of this information was being contradicted by top medical professionals. It did not help that the media literacy movement in schools was in its infancy, so most Americans were ill-equipped to determine what was truth and what was falsehood.

In the case of the great fart transmission theory, tabloid newspapers were among the first to promote the half-truth that farts were capable of carrying the virus in an airborne fashion and spreading the infection. An April 2020 edition of the British newspaper *The Daily Star* promoted the idea that Covid-19 was spreading worldwide through farts. The paper published an article with an erroneous headline, "Coronavirus 'could be spreading across the globe through farts' claim doctors." Only when readers got further down into *The Daily Star* account did it become apparent that infected people could "wear pants" to prevent this theoretically plausible form of virus transmission from occurring.[13]

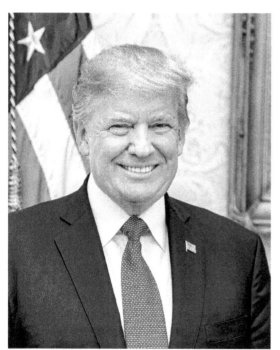

As president during the first year of the pandemic, Donald Trump created an atmosphere ripe for viral fart conspiracies with his assertions that Covid was no worse than the flu, that death rates were exaggerated, and that the virus would just disappear "like a miracle" one day (Library of Congress).

Media literacy experts decry the age-old tabloid technique of luring an audience into a story with a sensational headline and only later providing context that makes the story less dramatic or even erroneous. Social media has gone full bore with this technique, which is sometimes referred to as the use of "click bait." On the Internet, click bait is headline wording with the sole purpose of attracting attention and encouraging visitors to click on a link to allow all the content to show up on a web page.

It's very likely that Panera Karen received her information about viral transmission through farting via click bait content that was repeated on social media websites. Soon, Panera Karen and kindred spirits were dismissing masks and exclaiming to others: "You think that mask is going to protect you? You fart out your ass! You can smell it out of your ass! You think that mask is going to protect you?"

Medical doctors made the effort to correct and to clarify the misinformation spread in tabloid newspapers and on the web. They stressed the importance of social distancing, wearing masks, and taking safety precautions. Part of the formula for being safe was that no one should fart close to other people and no one should fart with a bottom bare in the vicinity of others. These advisories inspired comedians like Stephen Colbert to comment, "I'm hoping that's pretty much always the advice," in an episode of *The Late Show* on CBS.[14]

Colbert did go on to suggest that besides wearing pants, farting into your elbow might be another measure to reduce any chance of viral transmission via flatulence. Critics of Colbert's advice noted that farting into your elbow would not be advisable because of the body contortions required. And attempting to whip your elbow down quickly enough to catch a fart could cause some serious head injuries. "After all, your elbow is usually not as accessible to your butt as it is to your mouth, unless you are doing some kind of twisty yoga pose," noted Colbert.[15]

Farts have been maligned for centuries. They've been blamed for human misfortunes and all manner of historical calamity. The bottom line is that farting may, indeed, push out air and aerosol particles rapidly like coughing and sneezing. Nevertheless, undergarments and pants provide that same protection that masks do in the case of coughing and sneezing. As long as people use some common sense and courtesy, such as not exposing bare bottoms in public, there's no need to be concerned about a Covid-19 fart transmission conspiracy.

Sorry, Panera Karen. It's long since time for you to zip it, simmer down, and just be quiet about the nonsense that you have spread. Masks can protect you in a pandemic, even if you do fart out your ass … and you can smell it out of your ass. Keep your mask, your shirt—and your pants on. Especially, keep your pants on! The great Covid-19 fart transmission conspiracy proved to be an excuse for those looking for a reason not to be inconvenienced by having to wear a mask. The conspiracy and the excuses were, in fact, inexcusable. They ultimately resulted in higher rates of infection, transmission, and mortalities.

CHAPTER 2

Fanning the Flames
of Fart Conspiracies

The bizarre tale of Panera Karen, who perpetuated a frightening fart contagion theory during the pandemic of 2020, is not some isolated incident. Popular culture, folklore, and the mass media have always been ready to fan the flames of fart conspiracies. Farts have been blamed for disastrous wars, pestilence, and the actions of terrible dictators. Farts have taken it on the rim for global warming, climate change, and loss of ice at Earth's poles as well as for super storms and for wildfires at various global latitudes.

Farts are not simply the subject of bawdy humor and barroom jokes. Plenty of conspiracies have been hatched about their impact on historical events—and in a few instances, those conspiracy claims have considerable merit. Additionally, farts have found a place in folktales, fables, and mythology. Flatulence has inspired some of the fulminations behind pseudo-science as well as some of the fodder for legitimate scientific theory.

Science has given us a whole new perspective on the early days of the planet and the evolution of life. Scientific discoveries are revealing that long before dinosaurs may have been doomed by their own methane, and long before Neanderthals and Cro-Magnon hominids were all about fumigating the land, billions of one-celled organisms were engaging in primordial flatulence. These infinitesimally small creatures came to life hundreds of millions of years ago below the surface of the oceans. They still exist today beneath some of the same ocean floors where they first found life.[1]

The single-celled microbes live on a diet of decaying flora and fauna that sinks to the bottom of the oceans. After consuming this primitive diet, the microbes produce methane expulsions not unlike those of more complex, multi-celled creatures inhabiting the land masses above. These expulsions can accurately be called "micro-farts." They are relatively harmless when inert and in isolation. However, put trillions of micro-farts together, release them en masse in quick succession, and we have a problem, Scotty.

Fortunately, scientists assure us, all these micro-farts are relatively safe when they combine with icy cold water in dark depths and then stay put in the form of a slushy, frozen methane hydrate. The material stays locked in place in layer after layer of sediments far beneath the rolling seas. However, if these hydrates were to break free and surface all at once, our planet would be hit with unfathomable destruction with almost certain extinction of most life forms.

In his extraordinary poem "Fire and Ice," Robert Frost discussed the end of the world and speculated whether it would be destroyed in a conflagration of fire or frozen into lifelessness by a sheet of permanent winter ice. With the latest scientific information, Frost would now have to revise his poem to include the possibility of the world ending due to a giant methane bomb. The world would be consumed by the release of a giant, microbiological fart. To paraphrase Frost, "Some say the world will end in fire or ice, some say in methane."

So what might cause methane hydrate deposits to break loose at once to inundate planet Earth? Scientists hypothesize that the giant fart bubbles might be unleashed after the planet is hit by a massive asteroid or meteor shower. An enormous earthquake causing giant fissures in the ocean floor might also cause an unexpected methane release. Another dramatic destabilizing force could involve unprecedented volcanic eruptions beneath the oceans or might involve the force of simultaneous detonations from the world's nuclear arsenals.

Then there's the impact of climate change. A warming planet could release damaging methane from thawed peat and melting permafrost on Earth's surface. However, global warming could also loosen the methane hydrate material now locked in place in cold layers of sediments under the ocean floor. It has happened before. A massive explosion erupting from the ocean depths may have caused the worst mass extinction in Earth's history some 250 million years ago, according to U.S. geologists.

In a September 2003 issue of *Geology*, Northwestern University professor Gregory Ryskin contended that an extremely fast, explosive release of methane gas from the oceans may well have killed 95 percent of Earth's marine species and 70 percent of land animal and plants at the end of the Permian Era.[2] This cataclysmic event occurred long before dinosaurs lumbered about Earth expelling their own deadly methane. Long before the dinosaurs lived and perished, deadly methane bombs were ticking and waiting to explode.

Scientists have long wondered what caused the massive extinction of the Permian Era. Ryskin has calculated that prehistoric oceans could easily have contained enough methane to liberate an energy expulsion approximately 10,000 times greater than the world's entire nuclear weapons stockpile going off at once. "I do think that such eruptions will occur in the future, though perhaps not in the immediate future, and not on the same scale. I cannot predict the exact time or location. It is very important to start research in oceanography to identify methane deposits," Ryskin said.[3]

Other scientists agree. They make the case that it is vitally important to understand what occurred below the oceans in the Permian Era. They argue that humanity runs the risk of reproducing a similar gigantic discharge event from the deeps. That's because burning fossil fuels are warming the planet, and another methane discharge event may be even more severe than the one 250 million years ago if hydrate dissociation is triggered again.

It's humbling to think that the very existence of mankind may be under threat from trillions of micro-farts going off together, released in quick succession from an oceanic event, causing global havoc and destruction. Colossal releases of methane from Earth's nether regions may have ended past ice ages and made Earth inhabitable in previous planetary epochs. However, the next gargantuan methane release may not be so benign, and a clothespin on the nose will not save you.

Flatulence in Biblical Times

The Four Horsemen of the Apocalypse appear in the prophetic book of Ezekiel in the Old Testament. They are harbingers of war, famine, and pestilence, but they do not signal the terror of a giant methane bomb emerging from the oceans to explode in the face of humanity. In fact, not even one of the horsemen's steeds exudes an apocalyptic flatulence. Nevertheless, analysts of Old Testament writings do reference the frequent breaking of a mighty wind from somewhere on high.[4]

Jim Dawson, in his seminal work *Who Cut the Cheese?*, describes the many passages in the Bible from which allusions to flatulence, both figurative and literal, can be construed.[5] Dawson cites a constant emission of wind blowing across the lands of Egypt and Israel in the pages of both the Old and New Testaments: "And there went forth a wind from the Lord" (Numbers 11:31); "and with his mighty wind shall he shake his hand over the river" (Isaiah 11:15); "A dry wind of the high places in the wilderness" (Jeremiah 4:11); "We have been with child, we have been in pain, we have as it were brought forth wind" (Job 30:27).

Farts are said to have played a role in the Fall of Adam and Eve, as described in the Genesis story. The two innocents in the Garden of Eden took a few bites from the tree of knowledge and soon found themselves coping with God's wrath and itching from a very bad case of the green apple dirties. The Holy Bible remains as both a sacred book and an historical document of the early times of man. It chronicles some of the unique challenges early homo sapiens faced. Recent fart scholarship puts a new light on many of the biblical tales, from the story of Noah's ark and his boat full of flatulating animals to poor Jonah being propelled from the exterior of a whale after a three-day stay in the creature's stomach.

The Genesis story informs us that Adam and Eve were clueless after the creator breathed life into each of them. At first, they did not recognize their own nakedness. They were not aware of any need for clothing on a chilly day. They very likely were not cognizant of their own propensity for passing gas. All of this changed, of course, once they ate from the Tree of Knowledge.

Adam and Eve had been instructed by their creator to enjoy all the fruits of the Garden of Eden except for the fruit from one tree—the tree of the knowledge of good and evil. Just as curiosity killed the proverbial cat, curiosity killed the idyllic life that Adam and Eve had going in their lovely garden spot. Eve became curious about the forbidden fruit after a conversation with an evil serpent. The serpent has been likened to an agent of Satan or Satan himself.

The serpent tells Eve that she will become like God if she eats of the forbidden fruit and she will have her eyes opened to the truth. Eve takes a few bites and then persuades Adam to also take a few chomps of the enchanted apple. They both immediately realize their nakedness, make some fig leaf and animal skin coverings, and then go hide in the woods. An angry God subsequently finds the unhappy couple, lectures them on their disobedience, and doles out punishment. Adam will have to work forever; Eve will have to obey Adam and endure much pain in childbirth; and the serpent will be doomed to crawling on its belly and eating dust.

A few observations on the Adam and Eve story:

- There is an assumption that Adam and Eve are humiliated by the sight of their genitals when they first realize their nakedness. In truth, the two were probably more embarrassed by the sight of their backsides, especially after digestion issues involving Eden's green apples. Green apples are known to cause bloating, excessive gas, diarrhea, and apple peel skid marks on the back of the old loin cloth.
- A whole lot of finger-pointing happens when God asks for who is at fault in consumption of the forbidden fruit. Adam points at

Eve. Adam also then blames God for taking his rib and making a troubling companion whom he never really asked for in the first place. A resentful Eve shifts the blame to the smooth-talking serpent that talked her into savoring the green orb, a precursor of today's Granny Smith.

- The finger-pointing spectacle in the Garden of Eden continues today, even though the origin of the practice is not readily recognized. Flatulence releases like those that occurred in the first apple orchard often elicit the same kind of blame shifting as experienced by Adam and Eve: Who did it? Was it Adam? Or Eve? Or a lousy snake with a bloated belly crawling on the ground? Did the Devil make them do it?

The story of Noah and the great flood is another familiar biblical story that can benefit from the latest insights on the role flatulence has played in the lives of early man. In hindsight, the potency of the tale of Noah's ark is even more impactful with the new scholarship of fartology. Nothing illustrates the staying power of the Noah story in a more tangible way than the erection of an ark as part of the Creation Museum complex in northern Kentucky.

The Ark Encounter, which opened in 2016, provides an historical narrative of the flood story as part of an Evangelical-themed amusement park. The park includes a 510-foot long and 50-foot high replica of Noah's ark. There are plans to add to the park in the next decade with the construction of a Tower of Babel. The Ark Encounter offers a tour inside the giant boat and displays of animal compartments for the long voyage of the boat during the world's greatest flood ever authorized by God.

The controversial Creation Museum in Kentucky has a mission, in part, to persuade visitors that dinosaurs roamed Earth at the same time as the first man and woman found a home in the Garden of Eden. There is, however, absolutely no scientific evidence for this contention. What's more, the Old Testament makes no mention of dinosaurs in its many stories about the descendants of Adam and Eve. To be sure, there are serpents and sea monsters that surface periodically in the Good Book, but there is not one Stegosaurus, not one Brachiosaurus, not one Pterodactyl to be found.

Dinosaurs and the lizard kings known as Tyrannosaurus rex were non-existent in the time of Noah, but the religious attractions in Kentucky maintain that prehistoric animals existed as recently as 6,000 years ago. Despite the creation controversy, the one thing we can be sure of is that there were farts at the time of the Garden of Eden as well as an abundance of flatulence when Noah's ark sailed the flood waters.

In the Noah's ark story, an angry God finds the human race to be so depraved that he regrets his act of bringing them to life. He reportedly discovers humans to be so corrupted and violent that he resolves to wipe them from the face of the earth—and with them, all the animals. However, a few humans and a few animals catch a break when God recognizes that a man named Noah is a righteous fellow who is good with his hands.

God seems to have an excellent carpentry background, as he instructs Noah in great detail on how to build a huge boat. The vessel must be built with cypress wood that is to be coated in pitch. The boat must be 300 cubits long, 50 cubits wide, and 30 cubits high. A cubit is 1.5 feet or about 18 inches long. The boat is to have a lower, upper, and middle deck with a very wide door to accommodate many large animals. Noah commenced to use his skills to do everything just as God commanded him.

God told Noah to load his family up on the boat along with the creatures of the earth, male and female. Not long after the live cargo was loaded, the rains came and they continued for 40 days and 40 nights. The flooding eventually covered the mountains and raised the ark high above the earth. The flood waters did not recede for several weeks even after the terrible storms ceased. When it was finally safe to get off the boat, God made a covenant to never again use a flood to punish and destroy mankind. He vowed that henceforth, every time a rainbow appeared with a storm, the colors in the sky would remind man of His sacred promise.

A few observations are in order about the Noah's ark story:

- Although God's boat design and Noah's woodwork were exceptional, it must be pointed out that an ark without windows meant the long voyage was no picnic with all the flatulating animals. Most animals fart. Hyenas, hippos, and hamsters put out especially noxious gas and are seldom welcome on lengthy cruises.
- A visit to the Ark Encounter in Kentucky can provide visitors some insight into what it must have been like on a boat packed with animals. This is especially true if you happen to tour the Kentucky boat and are walking behind busloads of kids from religious schools. Whether they are secular or spiritual, children are known to give off scents that in no way mimic burning incense.
- Another issue to consider is Noah's own age problem. Biblical accounts estimate Noah's age at the time of the flood to be 600 years. This man could have been an AARP member for half a millennium and some change. Most old men begin to lose sphincter control in their 80s. Add Noah's flatulence to that of the hyenas, hippos, and hamsters. On the plus side for God's

chosen ship captain, Noah's age may have made the old sailor fart-tolerant—a major advantage considering his beastly cargo.

- Few people read through to the end of the biblical story of Noah, since it is anti-climactic and somewhat disturbing. After making a sacrifice to God for keeping him and his crew seaworthy for more than 40 days, Noah hangs one on by drinking copious amounts of vino. He also gets naked—not a pretty sight at age 600. But a tight loin cloth is murder when one feels bloated by the pleasures of the grape and after a long bout of seasickness. Noah's boys were embarrassed when they discovered Dad's condition after the cruise. They covered up his nakedness and vowed to keep his condition under wraps.

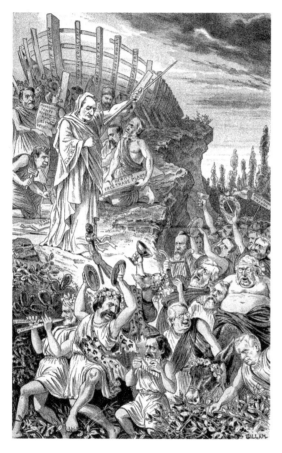

Scientists express skepticism over Old Testament stories such as Noah's ark, because a boat trip with wild animals of every species, farting together for 40 days and 40 nights, is simply not sustainable. The ark story has inspired political satire, such as this 1884 illustration by American artist Bernhard Gillam (Library of Congress).

Before taking leave of the amazing ark escapade, it's worthwhile to take another look at—or whiff of—the issue of hundreds of farting animals, male and female, on a boat. This problem of the extended aroma on the ark was somehow overlooked in the biblical account of Noah and his mind-numbing menagerie. This problem can best be put in perspective with an introduction to Nick Caruso and Dani Rabaiotti's work *Does It Fart? The Definitive Guide to Animal Flatulence*.[6] Their work analyzes in detail the "anal breath" of more than 100 prominent animal species alive at the time of Noah.

Besides examining the

flatulence of hyenas, hippos, and hamsters, *Does It Fart?* provides authoritative information on other animals that were corralled into the great ark of Captain Noah. Among those animals are lions, elephants, rabbits, and goats. Lions are almost exclusively meat eaters and thus producers of extremely pungent meat farts. Elephants eat tons of low-grade vegetation and are hind-gut fermenters, which makes them prolific and potent fart emitters. Rabbits must fart or die, so they fart often, according to *Does It Fart?* Goats have four stomachs full of methane-producing bacteria, so these bearded wonders added to the amalgamation of anal perfume on the ark.

Although scientists contend that dinosaurs disappeared from Earth more than 60 million years ago in a mass extinction event, the Ark Encounter experience in Kentucky insists that a variety of the large herbivores were in the queue to get on the good ship farty-pop. Many of these dinosaurs had digestive systems mimicking hind-gut fermenters like today's dwindling number of elephants. If the Creation Museum and the Ark Encounter are correct about the availability of dinosaurs for Noah's boat trip, then undoubtedly they contributed much of the flatulence on the floating refuge from a flood of biblical proportions.

The Ark Encounter site in Kentucky will reportedly add a novel Tower of Babel experience to the landscape of its biblical theme park.[7] An animated recreation of the David and Goliath story would certainly be a crowd-pleaser as well. The story of the young boy who took on a giant is one of the most popular and oft-repeated religious tales. It's the story of how a determined underdog can defeat a much larger opponent against all odds and has been used numerous times in sports analogies.

The Old Testament account of war between the Israelites and Philistines centers on the giant Goliath challenging any Israelite to a fight. If Goliath won, the Philistines would make the Israelites their servants and rule over them. If an Israelite was victorious, the defeated Philistines would become the subjects of the Israelites. The imposing Goliath stood more than nine feet tall in heavy armor and carried a huge spear. No Israelite chose to accept the challenge of the mighty warrior until David, a lowly shepherd boy, took up the dare.

David stepped out to face Goliath. He was armed with his slingshot and several smooth stones from a nearby stream, which he removed from his shepherd's bag. David called for the help of the deity of the Israelites, which angered Goliath. David then fired a stone from his slingshot. The potent pebble lodged in Goliath's forehead and brought him face down to the ground. David rushed the fallen giant and cut off his head immediately. King Saul rewarded the smallish victor with a place in his court and the Philistines were vanquished.

A few comments are in order on the victory of David over Goliath:

- Critics of the story contend that David was not such an underdog as portrayed in the Old Testament. In his *David and Goliath: Underdogs, Misfits and the Art of Battling Giants*, Malcolm Gladwell argues that size doesn't matter; it's the weapons of choice that make all the difference. David's slingshot was an effective military weapon that took out an opponent from a distance.[8] Goliath could not get close enough to wield his sword and slash David to pieces.
- Size may not make a difference, but diet does. The giant Goliath consumed great quantities of meat. Fattened oxen and sheep are high in protein but also cause sluggishness and they both take time to digest. In contrast, young David ate his veggies and was a lean, mean, slingshot-wielding machine with keen mind and quick response.
- Old age left the giant with poor eyesight. His eyes were reportedly watering at the time of his confrontation with David, exacerbated by meat fart flatulence and goat bloat. In context, a case can be made that this biblical battle was not a fair fight. Despite all assertions to the contrary, the giant was at a distinct disadvantage.

Another biblical tale involving a giant and a smaller being, with the important advantage of having divine providence on his side, is the story of Jonah and the whale. Despite its brevity, the story has found a place in literature and popular culture on numerous occasions. Allusions to the Jonah predicament of being swallowed by a whale exist in the literary classic *Moby Dick* as well as in cinema offerings such as Disney's film adaption of *The Adventures of Pinocchio*.

In this whale of a story, an angry God commands Jonah go to the city of Nineveh. Jonah must deliver God's foreboding prophecy against the inhabitants because of their great wickedness and insolence against their creator. Jonah proves to be a poor errand boy. Rather than carrying out the command, he joins sailors setting sail for Tarshish. The sailing ship runs into an unusually violent storm and the sailors determine that Jonah is to blame and so they throw him overboard.

Jonah barely has time to tread water before he is swallowed by a huge aquatic animal, presumably a whale, and he takes up quarters within its belly for three days and three nights. Jonah prays for an exit from the whale and he is spewed forth, whereupon he carries out God's directive to inform the inhabitants of their impending demise. The story gets more involved from there. God forgives Nineveh. Jonah appears resentful that he delivered a false alarm. Jonah and God have words after Jonah complains about sun exposure and his wish to die and be done with it all.

Suffice it to say, it's the story of three days and nights in residence in a whale that captures everyone's attention, not the account of Jonah's frustrations after he carries out the command of his heavenly master. In fact, the story of Jonah's lodging in the whale has had nature types scratching their heads for centuries. They ponder what kind of strange fish it was and scientists speculate on whether the fish story is even credible.

The story of Jonah and the whale may be the only biblical tale to undergo cross-examination in a court of law. In the famous Scopes trial of 1925, attorney Clarence Darrow questioned William Jennings Bryan regarding the literal truth. Darrow asked Bryan: "When you read that [in the Bible] … the whale swallowed Jonah…. How do you literally interpret that?"[9] Bryan responded that he was a believer in "a God who can make a whale and can make a man and make both of them do what he pleases." Bryan ultimately had to back off his literal interpretation of the Bible and was bested in the Tennessee courthouse contest by Darrow.

Scientists generally side with Darrow that the story of Jonah and the whale, while capturing imaginations for centuries, stretches credulity. In the harsh light of that skepticism, a few comments are in order about the giant fish swallowing Jonah:

- Scientists point out that while whales have large mouths, their throats are generally only a few inches wide. A man could not be swallowed whole. Only the sperm whale could conceivably swallow Jonah in his entirety. Sperm whales are notable for swallowing and digesting giant squids.
- Whales are incredibly large and produce enormous amounts of gas. Their methane fart bubbles are gargantuan and seafarers downwind from a whale fart report that when their bubbles surface and burst, the wind that breaks over the waters is extremely pungent.
- Although Jonah may have been swallowed whole and found himself in one of the sperm whale's four stomachs, he would not have lasted long because there would be no air or oxygen, only methane gas. What's more, the muscular walls of whale stomachs are used to crush food.
- The famous Bible story has the whale vomiting out Jonah after three days. Because of the small esophagus of the typical whale, it is more likely that Jonah was farted out from the other end of the whale. The huge methane bomb would have consisted of a giant fart bubble had the whale been submerged. Jonah might have had to surface inside a giant whale fart bubble.

Old Testament literalists may contend that the introduction of flatulence into the stories of Jonah and the whale, Adam and Eve, Noah's ark, and

David and Goliath constitutes a fart conspiracy in itself. Naturally, they might conclude that scholars of fartology are agnostics, atheists, or secular humanists. Literalists may be inclined to dismiss the flatulence interpretations as sordid attempts to diminish the credibility of the creation myth or as assaults on the veracity of stories about the divine power to flood the earth or assist in the killing of a giant. Nothing could be further from the truth.

Objections from American Evangelicals and the Creationists in Kentucky aside, the scholarship of fartology actually makes archetypal biblical stories all that more miraculous and awe-inspiring. The parents of the human race suffering from a case of the green apple dirties in the Garden of Eden? The release of an imprisoned Jonah via a giant whale fart bubble? Hundreds of animals noisily flatulating together in Noah's ark? All of this nitty-gritty serves only to bolster the literal realism of biblical stories and in no way denigrates them.

Flatulence Alters World History

Beyond putting a new light on biblical stories, the scholarship of fartology adds to our knowledge of world historical events. A few examples are offered here. These stories often intimate that the course of history was altered by flatulence. Further research into the details of the several examples offered here would tend to confirm this. History contains farts, but farts also can determine history.

Inevitably, some of the updated historical accounts—in the light of new information—are going to be relegated to the trash bin of historical fart conspiracies. That's to be expected in a world where fake news, doctored videos, disinformation, and unreliable social media have all increased skepticism exponentially. Nevertheless, more and more scholarly research is verifying any number of new "takes" and perspectives on historical events.

A fantastic fart event traced to ancient times has garnered coverage in such media venues as *Men's Health* magazine and *The Daily Beast*.[10] The incident in Egypt dates back to approximately 570 BC and involves a paranoid king named Apries. King Apries was worried about a revolt by his subjects and sent his trusted general Amasis to simmer things down. Instead, the mutineers befriended Amasis and enlisted him to be their new king. He was favorably disposed to this new assignment, much to the consternation of King Apries.

Subsequently, Apries sent a favored adviser to inform Amasis that his new role was not appreciated and that he should hasten back for a consultation with Apries. When the adviser confronted Amasis, the new royal turned his backside to him and released a defiant gassy message. Amasis told the messenger to deliver *this* message back to King Apries. As often happens, the king blamed the messenger for the insulting message and hacked off his ears and his nose. The brutality of Apries so enraged the Egyptians that they overthrew him, thus ensuring the official reign of Amasis from 569 to 525 BC.

Another startling flatulence event that resulted in violence involves an historic fart released during a celebration of the Jewish Passover in Jerusalem in 44 AD. This is sometimes referred to as the incredible "Gassover Fart." The incident resulted in the deaths of 10,000 people, according to the author Flavius Josephus in his account *The Jewish War*.[11] Josephus lived from 37 to 100 AD. He described the actions of a Roman soldier who bared his backside toward an assemblage of Jews celebrating the Passover.

As the Jews gathered to partake in festivities and to feast, the soldier standing watch above the temple revealed his bare butt and passed an audible insult upon the multitudes. The religious crowd reacted angrily to the blasphemy. Rioting erupted and the Roman soldiers rushed in to quell the disturbance. A stampede resulted that killed many of those celebrating the Passover. Jewish historian Josephus provided this account of the melee:

> The Jews' ruin came on, for when the multitudes were come together to Jerusalem, to the feast of unleavened bread, and a Roman cohort stood over the cloisters of the temple (for they always were armed and kept guard at the festivals, to prevent any innovation which the multitude thus gathered together might take), one of the soldiers pulled back his garment, and cowering down after an indecent manner, turned his breech [ass] to the Jews, and spoke such words as you might expect at such a posture. At this the whole multitude had indignation, and made a clamor to Cumanus (the provincial Roman procurator), that he would punish the soldier; while the rasher part of the youth, and such as were naturally the most tumultuous, fell to fighting, and caught up stones, and threw them at the soldiers.[12]

No emission of flatus has so directly resulted in such widespread mayhem and mass death as the so-called "Gassover Fart." However, it can be argued that discomfort and pain from chronic flatulence may have played a major role in German dictator Adolf Hitler's propensity for cruelty and mass violence. Alternately, it can be argued that Hitler took drugs for his flatulence that impaired his judgment and hastened the end of World War II. Hitler's many health problems with flatulence, and their impact on his behavior before and during the war, have been the subject of much historical research and debate.

Hitler suffered from what is known as meteorism, which is evidenced by the swelling of the abdomen from excess gas in the gastrointestinal tract. In his childhood, he suffered from excruciating stomach cramps. By the time he reached his 40s, the abdominal pain became more frequent with bouts of savage farting. He became a vegetarian, but he was still reportedly farting like a horse when he assumed leadership of Germany in the 1930s.

The Führer's intestinal ailments did not abate even with his conversion to a diet devoid of meat and dairy products. He did find some relief when he acquired a personal doctor after meeting Dr. Theodor Morell at a Christmas party. Morell was looked upon as a suspect pill-pusher and quack by respectable physicians. However, he remained Hitler's most trusted physician all the way up to the German leader's suicide in his bunker as Soviet soldiers entered Berlin.[13]

Pills that Morell prescribed for Hitler's bloating and flatulence literally began to poison him. At the same time, his malady worsened and he was known to fart noisily at dinners, stately events and in his war room. No one was so bold as to complain about Hitler's indiscretions, but Morell pushed more dangerous pills in Hitler's direction. Several of his generals were convinced that he was hallucinating, becoming more irrational, and manifestly losing his mind.

When tens of thousands of German soldiers were being surrounded by Russian soldiers at Stalingrad in 1943, Hitler was unable to think clearly and to agree to their evacuation. The surrender and loss of his Sixth Army was a turning point in the war and hastened its end. This is why some experts sur-

A credible flatulence conspiracy theory holds that Germany's Adolf Hitler was unable to think clearly at the end of World War II because of medicines he was taking for gas. Flatulence maladies were destroying his brain and poisoning him (Photofest).

mise that his flatulence, and the manner in which it was addressed medically, had an unmistakable impact on the outcome of the war.

More than 75 years after the death of Hitler and his Third Reich, historians and commentators continue speculating about the Führer's flatulence. Comedians crack jokes about "Adolf Shittler" and discuss his condition on late night entertainment shows. In 2019, comedian Jimmy Kimmel and history book writer Bill O'Reilly conversed about Hitler's final days. "Can you imagine, in the bunker, with Adolf?" O'Reilly asked Kimmel. O'Reilly suggested that the choice for those in the bunker was between inhaling Hitler's fumes or going outside and taking a bullet in the head as Berlin crumbled in defeat.[14]

The subject of flatulence in wartime has not been confined to discussions of World War II. After the terrorist attacks on the World Trade Center in New York City in 2001, American troops went into battle in Afghanistan and Iraq. The Afghan conflict, America's longest war, did not go well. In 2021 the troops came home and the Taliban enemy resumed control of their war-torn country in the Middle East. Flatulence may not have been to blame for America's failures in the Afghan war, but it certainly played a role.

Succeeding in a war halfway around the world is not just about besting enemies in armed conflict, it's also about winning the hearts and minds of "friendlies." If important allies are offended and alienated, then the mission can and will go south. American troops in Afghanistan racked up early successes in a war against the radical Taliban, but after 20 years of sacrificing blood and treasure, the United States left Afghanistan in 2021. The Taliban enemy took back control of the country within days.

What went wrong? Critics of American military strategy in the Middle East offer a number of hypotheses. Some explanations note the all-important factor of winning the hearts and minds of the locals. Americans went about their Afghan mission in blissful cultural ignorance of values important to Afghan natives. One of those important values involves flatulence.

For Afghans, nothing is more offensive than a shameful and arrogant exhibition of flatulence. Loudly passing gas is proof that a man is incapable of controlling all the functions below his belt, according to Afghan cultural standards. A man who revels in such behavior should not be taken seriously, nor should his assertions and pledges be considered reliable.[15]

When American commanders realized that farting by their troops was putting a cloud over the U.S. mission in Afghanistan, they put out the order to young GIs to end the culturally alienating, boyish pranks of ripping ass. Soldiers were asked to quiet their buttocks, to make friends with village elders, arrange to partake in traditional teas with locals. However, some young Americans could not resist in farting escapades, so much a part of their own culture back home. Never mind the Afghans offended by the behavior of the grunts, the grunts were offended by the directives of their commanding officers. Jarheads found it laughable that they were being told to defer to the sensibilities of a culture that they deemed primitive. The troops did not hold back.

When U.S. aircraft evacuated troops and friendlies from the Kabul airport in August of 2021, it brought a 20-year occupation to an end. Americans were upset that their long commitment would be remembered for ignominious failures, broken promises, and the spectacle of a frantic final exit. It all raised a stench. Part of that stench may well have been colossal misunderstandings over flatulence. In any case, the U.S. military abandoned a literal morass. The troops came home to where they could fart at will.

America makes dramatic history every four years with its presidential elections. This is especially true in a new century when two presidents lost the popular vote but attained the highest office through the Electoral College. George W. Bush lost the popular vote in 2000 by 543,000 votes. Donald J. Trump lost the popular vote in 2016 by 2,870,000 votes. In 2020, Trump made political history by refusing to concede an election he lost by more than 7,060,000 votes. To make the case that the election was stolen, Trump enlisted attorney Rudy Giuliani.

Known as the "nation's mayor" for his leadership of New York City after the 2001 terrorist attack on the World Trade Center, Giuliani suffered a precipitous decline in his stature and reputation during his legal battles on behalf of Donald Trump. The Trump campaign lost its bid to overturn the results of the election in courts across the country. Giuliani's credibility waned as his arguments became more untenable, as his hair dye had a meltdown in a press conference, as his ability to contain his gas was lost in a critical election hearing.

Classified as "squeakers," the farts were not only heard by those sitting beside Giuliani but were also picked up by courtroom microphones. Michigan Democrat Darrin Camilleri tweeted about Giuliani's toots, much to the consternation of the Trump attorney. Camilleri also testified about the tooting after late night TV host Jimmy Fallon mocked the former mayor of the Big Apple on his show, asking, "Can we go one week without something leaking out of Rudy Giuliani?"[16]

Politicians and attorneys have been known to emit gas on a fairly regular basis. Camilleri stressed that Giuliani's gas was emitted while using taxpayer dollars to investigate illegitimate claims of election fraud during the middle of a pandemic. He called it cowardly and cruel. The woman seated next to Giuliani was not so hot on his back-of-the-pants emissions either. Reporters noted the horror on attorney Jenna Ellis' face as Giuliani unambiguously cracked out a pair of stinkers. In Dublin, the *Irish Times* called his performance a "Reichstag moment." The Irish newspaper noted that Giuliani's co-counsel, Ellis, seemed to be giving her partner a grossed-out "dude, you beefed" look.[17]

A once-handsome, articulate prosecuting attorney in New York City, Giuliani looked like a tiny, faltering, political dinosaur in his final appearances before being relieved of his duties by Trump. Pundits wrote that Giuliani had crashed and burned. His efforts on behalf of Trump's "Stop the Steal" campaign seemed to run out of gas at a press conference that he filled with gas. Like the prehistoric dinosaurs, Giuliani was done in by his own methane.

Micro-Farts, Cows, Our Flatulence Future

Human farts have unquestionably altered the history of man. Dinosaur farts may have resulted in the extinction of entire species. Then there's the issue of bovine flatulence and its dire consequences. This chapter began with a discussion of an apocalypse that could result from the release of trillions of methane micro-farts locked in formations beneath the sea. All these micro-farts are relatively safe when confined as frozen methane hydrate below the oceans. However, they could be unleashed by warming waters from climate change. If all this methane breaks loose and surfaces at once, Katy, bar the door. Terrible destruction will ensue.

Scientists hypothesize that the great methane hydrate explosion is probably several centuries in the future. Forget the methane micro-farts from one-celled organisms for now; more worrisome are the macro-farts from multi-celled creatures known as cows. Global methane emissions from livestock farts are happening in the present. They are increasing in volume every year and entering the atmosphere to produce global warming. Methane from bovine farts is an especially destructive greenhouse gas and difficult to capture or neutralize.

For too long, concern over climate change has focused on the effects of CO_2 production rather than methane. Unfortunately, methane is approximately 30 times more effective in trapping the sun's heat than carbon dioxide. Carbon dioxide gets more attention because there is much more of this noxious gas and it hangs around much longer. Although CO_2 has a longer-lasting effect, methane has an impressive track record for warming in the near term—and a hefty percentage of today's warming is attributed to methane.[18]

Every cow expels in the neighborhood of 30 to 50 gallons of methane on a daily basis. This fact becomes all the more alarming with the realization that there are about 1.5 billion cows roaming the planet. A global herd of cows constantly belching and farting translates into big headaches for Mother Earth. *The Lancet*, an internationally trusted medical journal of clinical, public, and global health knowledge, recommends a dietary conversion toward plant foods and away from animal products.[19] A future of vegan and vegetarian diets could result in some of the greatest reductions of greenhouse gases.

The American medical profession has petitioned Congress and the White House to cut U.S. meat and dairy production in an effort to tackle the methane component in the current climate crisis. A new dietary template that relies more on plant-based foods, such as vegetables, fruits, whole grains, legumes, nuts, and seeds, can promote health while reducing environmental impacts.

Nevertheless, politicians who embrace the calls for fewer livestock farts, and more healthy diets for humans, can expect stiff resistance.

Opponents of a shift away from diets dependent on meats—with the noble goal of reducing mass livestock flatulence—have reacted cynically and just see a chance to make political hay. Trump White House aide Sebastian Gorka told the Conservative Political Action Conference in 2019 that "climate loonies" are a threat to the American lifestyle: "They want to take your pickup truck. They want to rebuild your home. They want to take away your hamburgers."[20]

Many right-wing politicians have joined in cries of "hamburger-gate." They insist that there's a left-wing, statist environmental movement that wants to end the ownership of cows, especially those of the farting variety—and they are all of the farting variety. Is there an insidious movement to end the American freedom to bite into a Big Mac, a Whopper, a Butter Burger or a White Castle slider? Will trumped-up flatulence hysteria end the era of the Big Boy, the Steakburger, and the Quarter Pounder with Cheese? Or is this all just another fart conspiracy?

CHAPTER 3

Farts Classified

Spiders, Ducks, and Squeakers

This study, and particularly this chapter, is in the tradition of founding father Benjamin Franklin, who was no stranger to writing about flatulence. He referred to it as "a stink in his breeches."[1] In a number of remarkable essays, Franklin speculated on such natural occurrences as human farting and the question of why such matters were not considered appropriate subjects for wordsmiths. After all, he suggested, "it is universally well known, That in digesting our Common Food, there is created or produced in the Bowels of human creatures, a great Quantity of Wind."[2] Franklin suggested that there was lasting damage in restraining that great quantity of wind. He surmised that suppressing farts caused pain, which probably resulted in ruptures, disease, and disagreeable demeanors.

Franklin was a scientist who was always trying to figure things out. In the case of flatulence, he concluded from empirical observation that most objections to its release could be attributed to the odiously offensive smells that accompany escaping gas. Franklin then began to investigate what foods produce the worst fetid smells and what foods might produce a pleasing air for which no one could raise objection. Franklin would likely take interest in the classification of farts in this chapter. Franklin wrote that dining on stale meat, accompanied by an abundance of onions, can be especially disagreeable for the nostrils in the aftermath. Referencing this study, it would be interesting to know whether Franklin might anticipate a "fire-in-the-hole" fart or a "rip-ass" fart after dining on stale meat and a mass of onions.

Franklin's unique observations on farting will be taken up later in this book. The object of this chapter is to produce a system of classification of the various species of farts that would make Carl Linnaeus *green with envy*. Past studies and scholarship on farting have always made the critical mistake of relegating glossaries of flatulence synonyms and terminology to the back pages. This is, quite frankly, half-assed backwards.

In order to intelligently think about, to write about, and to discuss the sometimes distressingly high incidence of farting, it's important to have a grasp of definitions and terms from the outset. The subtleties and nuances contained in such expressions as prostate poof, fizzler in the fundament, steaming duffy, and blue dart call out to be understood. This comprehension is not just clinically useful, it's entirely necessary. For example, a grasp of this terminology will be especially helpful in succeeding chapters when analyzing the plight of the various subsets of gas passers afflicted with a range of ailments.

1. **"Rip-Ass" Fart.** There is no mistaking the rip-ass fart. There is no mistaking the obnoxious sector of humanity that revels in releasing such aromatic chaos, often upon the innocent and unsuspecting. The fart itself is characterized by an unusual force of propulsion. The perpetrator has no interest in suppressing the bombast or in releasing the gas incrementally. Instead, there is a conscious effort to contain the odiferous outlay and to allow it to build up for maximum effect upon its departure. The entire operation with the rip-ass fart involves concentration on controlling the sphincter muscles to delay the launch until restraint is no longer tenable. Then the muscles are forcefully employed to propel the payload into the ether—or whatever expanse may be available.

The results of the ignition and liftoff are nothing less than spectacular for anyone in close proximity of the organic material's launch pad. Quite often there are audible groans and protests from miserable victims as well as physical manifestations of discomfort including watery eyes, salty lips and mouth, and conscious attempts to suppress normal breathing. The keyword here to describe the whole "rip-ass" phenomenon is "toxic." The sulfurous nature of this kind of emission brings to mind Environmental Protection Agency regulations to protect the public from toxic smoke stack venting or crusty drain pipe overflows. The brigand who relishes bringing this kind of pestilence upon the world is easily identifiable as a practitioner of toxic masculinity.

Boisterous, wild-eyed, heavy-set men are most often fingered as the unapologetic goons who are likely to perform the role of shameless rippers-in-chief. It's all about toxic masculinity. Toxic masculinity has been described as a male propensity to aggressively compete, to dominate, and to humiliate. In the case of the commission of a rip-ass fart, the chief aim of the nefarious activity is to establish an indisputable record for one of the most disgusting and disturbing acts of bodily malfeasance. The object also is to force all those in the immediate vicinity to suffer and absorb the airborne toxicity. The unfortunate casualties can be helpless captives in a moving car or sedentary souls confined to a classroom site. These are spaces where escape is not easily accomplished. There's a certain uncaring criminality in the perpetration of the rip-ass fart. The pity is that there are no laws on the books to protect society from this criminal behavior.

The rip-ass fart also is sometimes referred to as an ass flapper, as a barn burner, as a booty bomb, as a butt bazooka, as a baked bean explosion, as an atomic burrito, as a seismic blast, and as simply a stink bomb. No adequate synonym actually exists that is an equivalent for the ultimate masculine descriptive of "rip-ass fart."

2. **"Silent-But-Deadly" Fart.** The major characteristic of the silent-but-deadly fart is, in fact, its deceptive quietude, its traitorous illusion of tranquility, its lack of a proper introduction—its subversive silence. The silent-but-deadly fart shares much in common with another weapon of human origin, the silencer. This muzzle device reduces the acoustic intensity of a firearm or an air gun when it is discharged.

Most proponents of the weapons-grade silencer maintain that its purpose is to protect the hearing of shooters and other people who happen to be near the blast. However, silencers can never be disassociated from their original connections to espionage, assassination, secretive crimes, or military special operations use. Likewise, the silent-but-deadly fart has less to do with the well-being and health of the malefactor, or nearby associates, and everything to do with homicidal-like impulses, if not outright urges to inflict pain and annihilation.

Also known as the SBD, this fart is like poet T.S. Eliot's "fog that creeps on little cat's feet," but this is not a kitten we're dealing with—and this fart is described as deadly for a reason. An SBD does not permit time to take cover or to find an opportune escape route. Many times the dangerous SBD will be preceded by a wisp of virulent vapor that may be dismissed as a nasal false alarm, because it seems so unlikely for such heinous smoke and mist to enter into the midst of polite company. By the time the warning signal is determined to be an opening salvo of the real thing, there's no chance to flee from a virtual five-alarm flare-up of acrid assault. The little cat's feet that were ushering in a strange fog have suddenly transformed into feline paws with cheetah-like claws mercilessly digging into a floundering victim.

There's a tendency among some to pardon the perpetrator of the SBD because, after all, it's quiet and seems less deliberate than the atomic rip-ass fart. No one should fall prey to the delusion that an SBD conveyor is somehow less arrogant or unfeeling than the dispenser of rip-ass gas. Please, don't be naïve. Just watch for the Cheshire Cat grin that spreads across the face of the guilty party responsible for the surprise attack of an SBD. Just watch for signs of perverse joy on the visage of an SBD aggressor who takes so much satisfaction in pulling off the element of surprise.

In fact, there is much evidence to support the proposition that the SBD carrier is every bit as sadistic as the full-blown, rip-ass fart offender. Forgiveness should never be accorded the SBD criminal. Pardons, if granted at all, should be reserved for the embarrassed owner of the one-that-got-away fart, which will soon be under discussion.

The silent-but-deadly fart gestates and originates with every age group and all manner of genders. It is sometimes referred to as a sneaker squeaker, as a back draft, as a tongue-tied tootsie, as a power puff, as a fanny floater, as a muted monster, as a mum bomb, as a noiseless nasty, as a quiet quake maker, as a closed-mouth mischief, as a tight-lipped Lucy.

3. **"One-That-Got-Away" Fart.** One clear distinction between a silent-but-deadly fart and the one-that-got-away fart is that everyone is surprised by this emission, including the emitter. It comes from out of nowhere and is totally uncalculated and unintended. The decibel level of this bad boy ranges from barely audible to a clearly audible sound resembling an abused musical instrument such as a tuba. The noisome release causes much embarrassment and humiliation for the sad sack who gets caught in the involuntary act.

The one-that-got-away fart is a deal breaker, a career killer and a relationship destroyer. It can be interpreted as a crushing admission that emission creep is in the works, that involuntary flatulence is in one's future, that the bowels might soon be beyond any semblance of control. There is good reason to leave the scene of this accident, as soon as possible, without so much as an excuse, an alibi, or an explanation.

Those who succumb to disbursing a one-that-got-away fart come from all walks of life, but the worst devastation occurs for those who are in positions of authority and responsibility. The horror of the one-that-got-away fart can be seen on the shocked faces of the humiliated, whether those faces are owned by anxious politicians announcing their candidacy for office or nervous soloists about to launch singing careers. It can be seen on the wilted visage of the seminar leader whose trouser seams appear to be ripping after being introduced to his audience. It can be seen on the crimson cheeks of the head librarian who has just raised a finger to her lips to hush noisy patrons and then finds she is the

Air Swallowing Can Cause Gas

soon after a potentially flatus-producing meal.

Among those antidotes are:

• Activated charcoal. A treatment, purported to be 2,000 years old, activated charcoal now comes in large capsules and can be expensive.

• Simethicone. A popular over-the-counter gas chaser, simethicone counters stomach gas but reportedly does little for flatulence.

• Lactaid. Lactase has been extremely successful among milk lovers who are diagnosed as lactose-intolerant.

A new product on the market, heralded by AkPharma Inc. as "a social breakthrough in the human gas category," is Beano. AkPharma contends that when drops are added to the first bite of offending food, Beano will break down the gas-producing sugars and prevent bloating, gassiness and discomfort.

Gastrointestinal expert Eckrich said he believes that Beano, and other alternatives to elimination diets for treating flatulence, are probably only effective for a small percentage of gas producers.

In fact, Eckrich noted, all normal healthy people are gas producers. Studies show the average person releases about a quart of rectal gas a day, or approximately 13 or 14 expulsions of various magnitude.

Of those people with chronic gas, only about one-third have the

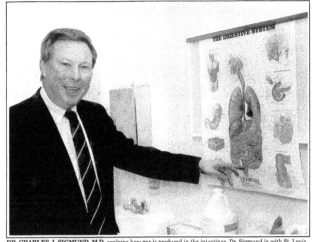

DR. CHARLES J. SIGMUND, M.D. explains how gas is produced in the intestines. Dr. Sigmund is with St. Louis Gastroenterology Consultants.   photo by Diane Dunham

Gastroenterologists are reluctant to classify farts as "rip-ass," "cheek squeakers" or "barking spiders." However, medical professionals such as Dr. Charles J. Sigmund of St. Louis, have pointed out the various causes for flatulence, ranging from dietary issues to motility problems (courtesy *Webster-Kirkwood Times*).

one shooting the breeze in the stacks. It can be seen on the crumpled forehead and averting eyes of the priest in the pulpit, when the holy of holies suddenly realizes his sermon has been permanently derailed by the staccato of an uninvited apparition.

So often, that cruel phrase "the one-that-got-away" is all about a lost love, about a lost romance, about what could have been if things had just worked out with that one special person. This often involves an unhealthy idealization, according to psychologists. It's pure fantasy about a past that never really existed. In contrast, the trauma of the one-that-got-away fart is real and not some lovesick fantasy. It involves an incident of an indelible nature that can scar for life. Go to a 10-, 25- or 50-year class reunion and there will always be the inevitable recollections of the poor girl who let one slip in algebra class; the speech teacher whose indiscretion of a mere three seconds will outlive any oratorical inspiration that she may have had to offer; or the double date at the drive-in theater that went south for everybody after the one-that-got-away filled the car.

The one-that-got-away fart has inspired a large number of synonyms that cannot be exclusively applied to one particular species of fart. The one-that-got-away fart is sometimes classified as a cheese doodle, as a hindquarters hiccup, as a corn slider, as a wall cloud, as a posterior peal, as a butt cough, as a prostate poof, as a fizzler in the fundament.

4. **"Whoopee Cushion" Fart**. Not all flatulence is about aggression, shocking incivility, and humiliation. Sometimes a short burp from the behind is simply an occasion for laughter among understanding friends. The whoopee cushion fart is most commonly emitted by those whom gastroenterologists have identified as air swallowers. This variety of emission is quite different than those prompted by digestion issues or difficulties with consumption of milk, meats, or beans. These emissions are deemed more acceptable, or at least more tolerable, because the fumes are less funky than those commonly associated with a rip-ass or a fire-in-the-hole fart. In other words, fewer protestations will be heard in the neighborhood because of this backside outrush.

The whoopee cushion fart brings forth an interesting chicken-or-the-egg kind of discussion. Which came first: the harmless fart that inspired the popular novelty item, or did the gag gift come first and then a certain genre of flatulence gradually acquired the moniker of "whoopee cushion" fart? This is one of those existential questions that may defy any definitive resolution.

The quandary is not unlike a related brain teaser: If a tree falls in the woods, but there's no one there to hear it, does it still make a sound? This begs an even more relevant question: If Jack Smart rips off a noisy fart in the woods, but there's no one there to hear it, does it still make a sound? These sorts of questions, like most philosophical dilemmas, are worth pursuing no matter how elusive the answers may be. Of course, one issue can be resolved easily without question: that the whoopee cushion gag gift has become a cash cow for the novelty industry.

The whoopee cushion is normally manufactured from two round sheets of rubber that are glued together at the edges. A small opening with a flap at one end allows air to enter and leave the cushion. When it is placed on a kitchen table chair, an unsuspecting victim is likely to sit on the whoopee cushion and then air is forced out of the opening. This causes the flap to vibrate to produce an embarrassing fart-like sound. Advertisements for these devices guarantee you will blow away your friends with the perfect prank toy. Another question to ponder: Has the ubiquitous whoopee cushion faux fart producer made the release of the real thing more acceptable in polite company—and if so, is that a good thing?

The real bona fide whoopee cushion fart is associated with a large number of synonyms that contain the words air, wind, breeze, and more.

Hence, it's not uncommon to hear this brand of flatus described as "breaking wind" or "baking brownies" or "beeping the horn" when a verb must be summoned. Nouns for this sort of activity include butt yodel, air biscuit, butt sneeze, trouser cough, trouser breeze, ass honker, butt hisser, hot wind, and fanny frog.

5. **"Cheek Squeaker" Fart**. The cheek squeaker is low in its decibel level and mild in its fragrance. The cheek squeaker merits little attention and often is not even acknowledged. When delivered in a library, few patrons will look up from the printed page or stop their Googling on a computer screen. When delivered in a restaurant, it is regarded as a mild annoyance at best and not an occasion to stop masticating or to halt the passing of condiments, the meatloaf, or the broccoli. The cheek squeaker merits discussion because it is so common, but also because there's a certain gender bias in labeling it as primarily a creation of the female sex.

At the risk of appearing sexist, casual olfactory analysts often make faulty assumptions such as categorizing the rip-ass fart as the exclusive province of the masculine posterior while classifying the cheek squeaker as feminine in nature. Also, experts assume that men pass the mustard much more often than women and that men produce more pungent odors. Not so. Sociologists tells us that women are more discreet with their gas passing, which is why they are typecast as cheek squeaker producers. Some scientists tell us that women's farts are actually more pungent than men's, but women are more likely to confine them to the bathroom and to give them time to dissipate therein.

Male comedians such as Howard Stern and the late George Carlin have made much of the so-called "lady fart," which is a vaginal air release totally disconnected from the digestive track production of the conventional fart. Carlin offered a notable, audible imitation of this strictly feminine release on his *Life Is Worth Losing* album. Stern has popularized this activity known as "queefing" on his radio shows. However, queefing should not really be confused with cheek squeakers. A final observation—the cheek squeaker gets a bit of play on a children's anime series that began appearing in 2014 on Japanese television titled *Yo-kai Watch*, which has featured a character with a butt-like face known as Cheeksqueek.[3]

Synonyms for the cheek squeaker fart tend to be non-descript and monosyllabic, which is not surprising given the nature of these puppies. Among the descriptive words in use are a blurp, a blurt, a pip, a putt, a thurp. Two-syllable expressions in use are boom-boom, drifter, floater, tootsie, frumper, rumper, and pop tart.

6. **"Duck Call" Fart**. This foul production is defined as a somewhat noisy, prolonged release of wind, which includes a quacking noise similar to a hunter's duck call. An actual hunter's duck call starts high and comes down the scale gradually with a rapid sequence of short notes, varying in pitch to mimic the sounds of ducks quacking. A proficient duck call fart practitioner will be able to vary the pitch of the production to suit the needs of any intended audience. Just as a duck hunter will be able to blow on his KumDuck device and tailor the calls for mallards, divers, or gadwalls (the most prevalent big duck in Louisiana), an experienced duck call farter can confidently croon a wide range of tunes for any assemblage.

No one has been more effective at popularizing the duck call fart, and bringing attention to its presence in American culture, than the late humorist and Hollywood actor Rodney Dangerfield. Dangerfield brings it all home in a marvelous scene in the 1978 classic movie *Caddyshack* when he holds court in a fine restaurant with a distinguished coterie of guests. In this favorite of golf cart cultists, Dangerfield is observed lecturing his table guests about investing in the stock market or real estate when suddenly he leans to one side to allow for the call of the backwoods. It's a staccato backfire that has his face wincing. When he tries to recover, he notices that the restaurant has become totally silent and filled with mortified glances. It's at this point that he blurts out the immortal line: "Oh, did somebody step on a duck?"

What's good for the goose is good for the gander and literally millions of people have appropriated Dangerfield's duck retort about his startling wildfowl flatulence for their own use. The line is employed by passers of the one-that-got-away fart to try to shift the blame for an odorous indiscretion onto someone else. The line is used in jest by the purveyor of the rip-ass fart. Dangerfield's line is a favorite of golfers in the clubhouse to show other hackers that they can be game for a bit of humor. Anyone who has witnessed the scene where Dangerfield coined the duck fart phrase will understand his other famous one-liners, such as "When I played hide and seek; they wouldn't even look for me" and his signature phrase "I don't get no respect!"

The duck call fart has naturally inspired flatulence synonyms that are related to animals or wildlife such as the reverse turtle, gopher grunt, bearded dragon, pupfish pewie, seal cyanide, hippo hiccup, sloth slider, wombat whisperer, clam chowder, squid rid, skunk squirt, bat skat, badger burp, and cheetah churro.

7. **"Barking Spider" Fart**. Men have used farts to taunt, test, and torment women from caveman days. Many young men are still as

primitive as cavemen and will trap their fair ladies under the covers—a practice known as the Dutch oven test. The captive damsel is smothered in the oaf's flatus, and if she endures the offense with humor, she passes the test of love, good-heartedness, and loyalty. A less toxic, but certainly an annoying practice, involves the male who continually farts and persists in asking his significant other: "Did you hear a barking spider?" The correct answer 100 times a day is yes, she did hear the bark of the spider. It's another test of love and loyalty. It's rude, but not as vulgar as being put in a Dutch oven.

A July 2007 post on the website Metafilter.com titled "I'm Dating the Barking Spider" reveals just how annoyed women can get with the woofing arachnid routine. She complains that her boyfriend farts in restaurants, in movie theaters, at concerts, at soccer games, everywhere. "They're not little amusing farts, but loud, long, malodourous farts.

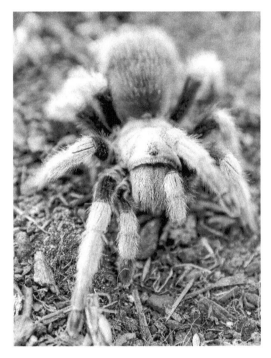

He and I both pretend like nothing's happened, which is hard for me because everyone around us is acting otherwise. Now when I go out with him I'm consumed with anxiety, wondering when he's going to let one loose. My attraction to him is waning. The last few times I went out with him I was overcome with revulsion."[4] More relationships have died in the Dutch oven and in the web of the barking spider than we will probably ever know. Sociologists have passed on researching this topic.

Those familiar with the barking spider fart may be surprised to learn that an actual barking spider exists Down Under. The Australian arachnid is a large, hairy tarantula that makes a kind of barking noise by rubbing rows of

In addition to being a type of fart, a "barking spider" is an Australian arachnid, a member of the distinctively hairy tarantula family. The aggressive Aussie spider has large fangs and makes a barking noise, much like a fart, to scare off any would-be predators (photograph by Ursula Ruhl).

its spines on its palyps, the appendages it uses to hold its victims. The barking noise wards off the spider's own predators. The barking spider is an ancient resident of Earth, and it has been sucking the life out of insects, birds, and frogs for eons. However, in more recent times, the barking spider moniker has been adopted by rock bands, such as the Australian group that put out the *Barking Spiders Live: 1983* album. Sports teams also have popularized the barking spider both inside and outside of the locker room. Denver's Rocky Mountain Rollergirls have championed a team member known as the Barking Spider, who "came into this world full of rage and farts."[5]

No synonyms exist that can approximate the term "barking spider." Obviously, some terms are in circulation that are loosely related to the barking spider. Among those expressions are monkey trumpet, dog smog, queefy walrus, butt bloviator, poof daddy, dog chime, ass droid, crank bug, daddy dingle berry, brown release, black widow, and stool loser.

8. **"Green Apple Dirty" Fart**. Also known as the "drizzler," the green apple dirty is one of the most feared farts among gas passers. This is because such an event can require a quick exit from any premises for a needed change of shorts, briefs, underpants, undies, underwear, or related undergarments designed to cover the rumpus area. The operative word here is *soiled*, as in the sincere expression of regret: "You must excuse me. I fear I have soiled my rompers." The ultimate regret with these incidents is when there is no real opportunity for a no-dalliance departure in order to retreat from the pant porridge disaster and to recover with a complete change of pantaloons.

Plenty of gas passers have had the most unpleasant surprise of thinking they are releasing a conventional fart only to find that they are unleashing the first salvo of the onset of diarrhea. The infamous brown highway in the caboose section of one's shorts is not always an indication of the presence of green apple dirties. However, there is no mistaking the eruption of a diarrhea attack within one's skivvies as anything other than a green apple dirty extended flatulence event. When there is no opportunity to change clothes in these situations, the best option is to seek out an 1800-watt hairdryer in the closest bathroom of your host. When on the road, seek out an Excel or Dyson hand dryer in a public restroom at the nearest rest stop. Do not attempt to drive more than 100 miles when the backside feels wetter than an otter's pocket.

From an historical standpoint, farm boys in 1800s America were known to complain of cramps, diarrhea, and soiled bib overalls after partaking in an excessive number of less-than-ripe green apples.

American foot soldiers serving in World War II in Europe were reportedly hampered by the green apple dirties as they advanced eastward to vanquish the enemy. Soldiers captured and held as prisoners of war suffered extended bouts of the green apple dirties from common amoebic gut infections.

Among the many euphemisms employed to indicate a case of green apple dirties are sputnik, nuking the fridge, yak shaver, back peddler, Georgia rose, soy sauce, sorority squat, fraternity condiment, wallpaper job, apple knocker, Hershey squirts, and TSIF, which can be an acronym for Transport Stream Interface, The Sky Is Falling or This Space Is Filled.

9. **"Fire-in-the-Hole" Fart**. Let's lay it on the line when it comes to this fart. It's an out-of-body experience that can result from a dinner that kicks off with jalapeño poppers, moves on to chili and beans, a full rack of spicy barbecued ribs and onion rings, followed by a late evening of golden lagers chased by tequila shots. The next morning's lethal hangover will inevitably be accompanied by flatulence that has the injured party yelling "fire in the hole!" This is probably the only fart in which the perpetrator suffers far more from the offense than those unfortunate enough to be near the white-hot expulsions.

An entire book could be written about the fire-in-the-hole fart, which derives its name, in part, from the intense pain and itching in the flatulence release area. This is an anatomical region where it is simply not polite to relieve an itch in public. The flame in the fundament is not so easily extinguished. This inflammation is only exacerbated by the ingestion of the kind of foods that cause intestinal mayhem, especially the tomato-based products of Italy, the curry offerings of India and Pakistan, the jalapeño dishes of Mexico, the jerk chicken of Jamaica, or the fire chicken of Korea. It's all about global mayhem.

The first cries of "fire in the hole" did not actually originate with the bombast of a fart so richly accented with a mist of spicy seasoning. The frantic cries of warning were originally used by miners to alert other miners that an explosive detonation was imminent, sometimes because of a build-up of combustible gases in the mineshaft. The fire-in-the-hole catchphrase also has been used in NASA's space program to signal the igniting of the upper stage of a rocket aloft, just as the spent lower stage is ejected. Fire in the Hole also is the name of a popular ride at Branson, Missouri's Silver Dollar City amusement park. The dark-themed roller coaster treats riders to fiery scenes. They are based on the historic burning of an Ozark town by a vigilante group known as the Baldknobbers.[6]

Related terms for the fire-in-the-hole fart include fart-ache, white hole, cactus fart, roasted rim, rim shot, spicy meatball, peppery poot, fire rhea, blister bum, roast beefed, hot pocket, cheese bubbler, burnt bowels, burnt popcorn, torrid tooter, dill hole, belching waffle, the brown growler, ring of fire, ash hole, steaming duffy, pencil sharpener, devil's nacho nest, browned round, catch twenty-poo, mud dungeon, and dirty tyler.

10. **"Methane Bomb" Fart.** The methane bomb fart harkens back to the rowdy college fraternity house behavior of the 1970s, which is perhaps best portrayed in the 1978 movie *Animal House*. Frat boys have a reputation for taking pride in personally fumigating their Tau Kappa Epsilon or Beta Theta Pi fraternity houses, then raving to their frat brothers about the launch of a methane bomb fart. Methane is among several gases including hydrogen, carbon dioxide, and hydrogen sulfide that all combine in the large intestine to give the fart its disturbing aroma. At some fraternity houses, the launch of a powerful methane bomb could increase a member's chances for election to the high offices of Grand Hegemon or Grand Prytanis.

Another practice popular with fraternity brothers and young male pranksters involves lighting a methane bomb fart. In order to ignite such a fart, it's necessary to have a lit match or a lighter near the rectum and to light up the flatulence as soon as it begins escaping. The resulting flare has sometimes been described as a "blue angel," a "blue dart," or "blue flame." Orange or yellow flares also are possible depending on the mixture of gases formed in the colon. The methane bomb flaming blue dart fart has been praised as a vehicle for male group bonding, but lighting up an emerging fart also has been condemned as stupid and a dangerous stunt that can cause serious injury.

Descriptive words or phrases capturing the essence of the methane bomb fart are many. In fact, some of the terms for the fire-in-the-hole fart also have application for the methane bomb fart and can be quite apropos. Among the most frequently used methane bomb equivalents are dank-worth, blue dart, trick fart, scorched berth, bowel howl, stinky winky, poop nuke, fecal fireball, morning thunder, meat grenade, goose pudding, combustible bunghole, tile peeler, and atomic sludge.

Four decades after National Lampoon's *Animal House*, college students seem to be far less interested in lighting up their methane bombs and more concerned about reducing the actual release of methane into the atmosphere. The reason for this concern is that methane has been identified as a potent greenhouse gas causing global warming, climate change, and an uncertain future for the planet.

Methane gas from human flatulence is just a fraction of the problem, however. Cow farts and bovine belches are far greater contributors to climate change. "That's because 1.5 billion cows across the globe are each expelling from 30 to 50 gallons of methane bombs every day."[7] Humans, who release their own methane bomb farts, can't really hold a candle to the rear end of a cow or the environmental damage that cows are causing.

CHAPTER 4

Tormented Gas Passer

Know Thyself

From Thanksgiving Day to New Year's Eve, Americans are famous for overindulging with major bouts of drinking, eating, and extreme merriment. On Thanksgiving, there are turkey breasts and drumsticks to devour along with endless bottles of wine for toasting and guzzling. Don't forget the candied yams and pools of rich gravy in reservoirs made of lumpy mashed potatoes or the desserts of minced meat, pecan, and pumpkin pies. Grab the silverware and let the spooning, slicing, and stabbing begin. It's time to give thanks and get stuffed with gooey stuffing and every other fatty side dish known to man.

For New Year's Eve, many eaters count on snack foods, including Flamin' Hot Cheetos, hot chili and lime tortilla chips, onion and garlic potato chips, and Hot Cheese Curls. Maybe the party to usher in the new year is more upscale and sports spicy hors d'oeuvres like jalapeño poppers, red pepper chicken wings, hot cheddar mini-muffins, jalapeño shrimp salsa, bacon-wrapped chicken livers, cranberry hot wings, or spicy peanut chicken wings. In any case, all this edible insanity is invariably slammed down with that famous combination of spirits enshrined in the American psyche by singer George Thorogood—copious amounts of bourbon, whiskey, and beer.

One of the undesirable after-effects of holiday stress and eating to excess is the discomfort of severe bloating. The bulging, ballooning feeling of abdominal cramps eventually gives way to an extended period of fart emissions. Sometimes the unwanted flatulence eruptions lead to embarrassing exhibitions. These can result in alienation of close acquaintances, in severance of family relations, and in lasting marital discord.

Doctors who specialize in gastrointestinal disorders agree that of the three major causes of gas passing outbursts, the easiest one to address is that involving consumption of mass quantities of food, such as items that are notorious for causing flatulence. Doctors readily identify these troubled gas-passers as humans whose digestive tracts resist the process-ing of beans, vegetables, and various legumes. Troubled diners also can suffer disastrous effects from ingesting hearty portions of red meat. Medi-cal experts can prescribe changes in diet for this gas-passing constituency for salutary effect.

More problematic than the troubled eaters category is that of the helpless air swallowers who in the extreme can bloat painfully like swol-len whoopee cushions—until some venue of relief can be found. That air must go somewhere and it does, indeed, find a final exit. The air swallow-ers have a condition known as aerophagia and it sometimes can occur in people with psychiatric conditions such as excessive anxiety or depression. Obviously, medical experts cannot simply prescribe dietary changes for this gas-passing constituency to achieve a salubrious outcome.

Finally, there is a third gas-passing constituency that is commonly plagued with motility issues or irritable bowel syndrome. These are the poor souls—some of whom are on the verge of becoming actual souls in the afterlife—who suffer the consequences of sluggish motility or irritable bowel. Their problems can include chronic constipation and fecal impac-tion. The poop is just not moving. Such problems can involve a complex interaction between the nerves and muscles of the intestinal tract and the regions of the brain that cause the sensation of pain. Medical experts can prescribe laxatives and enemas, but these don't always get the job done and are not satisfactory solutions.

Most members of the human race regard their flatulence as an occa-sional social inconvenience. Some may actually find enjoyment in the ability to drop a methane bomb or unleash a barking spider in selected company. However, many victims of troublesome farting ask questions and seek solutions to their problem. They are uncomfortable just sitting on the problem and simply wishing it to go away. This chapter may open some of the doors of perception and enlightenment for those who fervently desire to know the "why" and "how" of addressing stubborn flatulence. This is all to the good. To paraphrase Socrates: "Gas passer, know thyself."

Full Meal Deal Flatulence

Gastrointestinal physicians around the world emphasize that the abnormal person is the one who doesn't fart. All normal healthy people are regular gas producers. Many are silent producers who may not even be aware of how they are contributing to sullying the atmosphere. Stud-ies show the average person releases about a quart of rectal gas a day or approximately 12 to 15 expulsions of various magnitudes. Releasing more than a score of farts daily can be a worrisome sign. Also, excessively aromatic farts can indicate that something has gone seriously astray.

Dr. David Armstrong, a professor in the division of gastroenterology at McMaster Medical Center in Hamilton, Ohio, draws on the wisdom of Chinese medicine in regard to flatulence. Armstrong notes that farting is one of the "three jewels" in Chinese medical understanding.[1] The other two are crying and sweating. Crying is an indication that the emotional system is functioning well. Sweating can be a sign that immune system is functioning properly. Farting is an indication that the digestive system is on the job with "all systems go."

Armstrong does caution that the average fart should not really smell all that much. Because most North Americans do not eat enough fruits and vegetables to keep things moving in their digestive systems, their farts can be unusually smelly to the point of appalling. Poisons like alcohol and certain junk foods also can cause alarmingly stinky gas. However, some very healthy foods also are capable of raising a stink after being ingested. Diet can be pivotal for what happens in the gut of the profligate gas passer.

The normal gastrointestinal (GI) tract actually contains only a small amount of gas, estimated to be 100–200 milliliters (about a cup). This increases to more than 300 milliliters following certain meals.[2] Some of this gas may come from swallowing air during eating, however, the majority is from gas production from metabolism of food products. Medical experts point out that in normal subjects, nitrogen, oxygen, and carbon dioxide are the predominant baseline gases with hydrogen and methane content kicking up after meals.

These gases distribute between the stomach, the small intestine, and the large intestine, known as the colon. The colon accounts for most of the normal gas content in the gastrointestinal tract. This gas is primarily the result of metabolic activity of the individual's gut microbiome—the bacteria that normally reside in our colon. The gut microbiome, by the way, has become an active area for recent research. The gut microbiome is defined as the community of microorganisms—bacteria, viruses, and fungi—that inhabit our intestinal tract, mainly the colon. The gut microbiome is a "community" that is not always at peace with itself.

There are more than 100 trillion individual organisms in the GI tract, made up of 1,000 different species. Taken together, these "bugs" harbor more DNA than we have in all our cells combined. Not only that, but they also help "define" the individual with whom they take up residence. There is less than 1 percent diversity between the DNA of all humans, despite our enormous variation in size, appearance, and demeanor. However, our gut microbiome DNA is very different from one individual to another and accounts for 80 to 90 percent of human diversity. It can be said that we are more the product of our gut microbiome DNA than of our own cellular DNA.

Scientists are just beginning to discover the many functions that the gut microbiome plays in health and disease, and flatulence is a big part of the mix. Among the many normal functions of the gut microbiome is the digestion of complex sugars and interaction with the immune system to help protect humans against disease-causing pathogens. It is no surprise, then, that when something perturbs the normal microbiome, then a variety of nutritional issues, GI disorders, immune regulation difficulties, and even problematic behavioral patterns result.[3]

Back to the issue of diet, most humans can become aware of particular foods that will result in gas production in their particular case. Common offenders include legumes, which are beans, soybeans, peas, peanuts, and lentils, to name a few. Although high in dietary fiber, and usually classified as health foods, they are also a rich source of nutrition for the gut microbiome. The bacteria use a breakdown process called fermentation in which complex sugars are metabolized to make short chain fatty acids and gases. These gases are mainly hydrogen but also carbon dioxide as well as the odoriferous gases like hydrogen sulfide and methanethiol.

Many people are aware of this breakdown process such as when yeast is used as a breakdown mechanism to produce alcohol. Normally, the excess gas in the breakdown process in the gut is not a significant cause of discomfort or concern. However, there are people who are plagued by excess gas and flatulence after a meal heavy in legumes. Other offending foods can include red meat or eggs, not necessarily resulting in excess gas, but in the production of the foul-smelling hydrogen sulfide or methionine.

A serious conundrum in our society is that as diets get healthier, the gas gets smellier. This may be due to increased intestinal gas from fermentation—or it may be that people are becoming more aware of this side effect. When actually measuring the number and volume of farting episodes in patients complaining of excess flatus, researchers may find that the number of episodes was within the normal range.[4] This is not to say that no one gets excess gas from a high-fiber diet, but the perception is often worse than the reality.

Obviously, for those who note excessive farting on certain diets, it is wise to consult health care providers to test for specific food intolerances. Same advice goes for people who have associated symptoms, such as bloating, pain, or changes in bowel habits. For the majority of people who just notice a little more gas with beans, there are methods to enjoy the health advantages of a high-fiber diet without feeling a need to stay isolated at home after meals. For those who enjoy going out and flaunting their flatulence, isolation at home is not really even a consideration. They're out to let it rip.

Remedies for excessive farting from diet include specific food eliminations through experimental consumption of one food item at a time to identify a particular offender. Is the perpetrator a spicy late evening snack, such as chili tortilla chips or jalapeño pretzels? Is the terrible culprit Aunt Martha's three-bean salad? Is the boogeyman the boiled cabbage accompaniment in a favorite Irish dinner? Do those beans doctored with brown sugar, molasses, and spicy barbecue sauce constitute a habitual summer offender?

Dieticians often recommend pretreating legumes by steaming or boiling them to reduce gas content. And, alternatively, there are specific diets that will eliminate the gas-forming fruits and vegetables while substituting those that are better tolerated. For people with specific food intolerances, there are over-the-counter digestive aids such as lactase in Lactaid or alpha-galactosidase in Beano.

Activated charcoal is another treatment purported to be more than 2,000 years old. Activated charcoal comes in large capsules and can be prohibitively expensive. Simethicone is a popular over-the-counter gas chaser to counteract stomach gas, but it reportedly does not always address flatulence. There is no panacea for fart problems that can have many different causes. There is no cure-all. Suffice it to say in regard to unwanted sulfuric aromas, the longer it takes for your body to digest food, the more time bacteria has to make some nasty odors when gas is passed in public. Chowing on high-fiber food and drinking lots of water will decrease the time that gas hangs out in the colon, causing less obnoxious odors, if that is a personal goal.

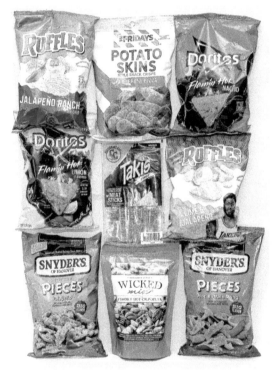

Jalapeño pretzels, chili tortilla chips, hot buffalo wing bites, and other spicy snack foods are loaded with saturated fat and salt, which can cause painful bloating and the nuisance of abundant flatulence (photograph by Ursula Ruhl).

In the final analysis, simply be careful about those large helpings of cruciferous vegetables, even though they are very healthy for human consumption. Among the gas-producing veggies are broccoli, cabbage, cauliflower, collard greens, mustard greens, radishes, rutabagas, and turnips. Be aware that a fatty filet mignon with sautéed mushrooms or a prime rib with plenty of horseradish can also trigger serious aromatic upheavals. Be nice and considerate of your gut microbiome. And always be wary of the Jerusalem artichoke. Known as "sun-choke," these little devils are a starchy edible root. There is a good reason seasoned gardeners and professional chefs call it the "farti-choke."

Air Swallowers Lament

We all swallow air every day, most often in connection with eating or drinking. Gulping down air during these activities is termed aerophagia. It also occurs with talking, laughing, chewing gum, smoking, and drinking carbonated beverages. In recent years, it has become an annoying side effect with the increasing use of CPAP machines. CPAPs may reduce snoring and sleep apnea, but they also can pump air into the body. Finally, unwanted air intake also is found among those who are sometimes referred to derisively as mouth breathers.

In a U.S. survey on gastrointestinal disorders, almost 25 percent of Americans admitted to occasional air swallowing.[5] From a practical standpoint, the absolute amount of air swallowed is rarely enough to cause discomfort or bloating. The majority of the air is simply belched back up through the mouth or absorbed by the body. However, some people are afflicted with flatulence when the air passes through the GI tract and subsequently is emitted through a lower aperture as anal flatus.

Significant aerophagia usually only occurs in people with associated psychiatric conditions such as extreme anxiety, depression, or cognitive delays. Some rare cases of aerophagia have been associated with neurologic injury. A review from the Mayo Clinic studied and characterized 79 patients with aerophagia between 1996 and 2003. The analysis found that about 20 percent suffered from anxiety. Associated symptoms included abdominal pain and abdominal bloating. Occasionally, severe flatulence was a result.[6]

In any case, a fundamental question remains. Do you suffer from aerophagia?

- You may have aerophagia if you have a habit of chewing gum and smacking vigorously or you suck on hard candies. These common habits will sometimes result in unnecessary air intake. More often than not, the excess air will find its way out of the body through belches and burps. However, if it does not find a way out through the way it came in, it's highly likely that flatulence will occur. Medical professionals will advise reducing or eliminating the use of gum and hard candies. Stop all non-essential chewing and sucking.

- You may have aerophagia from talking excessively while chewing on food or gulping down meals in a hurry. This can be exacerbated when the meals are accompanied by carbonated beverages such as soda or beer. Bubbly liquids naturally generate excess gastric air. Medical professionals will advise a reduction in such drinks and will also urge patients to have a calmer and quieter demeanor at meal time. Stop the unbridled blabbing.
- You may have aerophagia from the effects as well as the remedies for sleep apnea. The disease of sleep apnea often requires a device known as a CPAP machine. The acronym CPAP stands for continuous positive airway pressure and it's a therapy machine for treatment of obstructive sleep apnea. The CPAP equipment uses a hose connected to a mask or nosepiece to deliver constant and steady air pressure to help you breathe while you sleep. This prevents the constant disruptions of sleep that lead to serious health issues. However, if the device's air pressure is not correctly calibrated for your needs, or if there are problems with the mask fit, aerophagia can result. Medical professionals will suggest that sleep disorder experts adjust your CPAP equipment. Stop the excessive air swallowing by getting your machine tweaked.
- You may have aerophagia if you are a mouth breather. There are numerous serious health consequences involved for those favoring the mouth, rather than the nose, for breathing. Among those undesired effects are dryness of tongue, teeth, and gums resulting in bad breath, gum disease, and tooth decay. Increased intake of germs, irritants, and bacteria can occur. Another problem for mouth breathers can be abdominal pain and discomfort from air swallowing. Medical professionals can explain the many ill effects of mouth breathing but can also provide health-improving remedies. Stop and close your mouth; start using your nose.

It should not be surprising, given the many causes for excessive air swallowing and flatulence, that the remedies also are numerous and variable. The majority (87 percent) of aerophagia patient problems have been addressed by doctors through behavioral treatments or the prescription of appropriate medications including an antacid, an anti-gas, an anti-spasmodic, or a lactase. As suggested by the review of patients in the Mayo Clinic study, the best treatment is avoidance of the activity or behavior that leads to excess swallowing of air. Only that will tell whether excessive flatulence was due to the air swallowing.

We all ingest some air when we talk, eat, or laugh. We are not going to totally stop talking, eating, or laughing for fear of farting. People with aerophagia just happen to gulp so much air that it produces uncomfortable gastrointestinal symptoms. A fart produced from air swallowing can sound just as loud and as obnoxious as a fart produced by diet intake or by constipation issues. In deference to the air-swallowers and their flatulence, their farts are

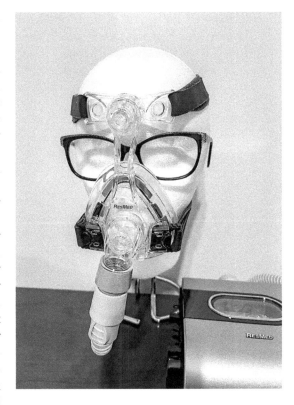

CPAP machines blow continuous air into nasal passages to address snoring problems and sleep apnea. However, CPAP air pressure can also cause aerophagia, which is excessive flatulence due to abnormal air swallowing (photograph by the author).

likely to be less odoriferous. In some cases, these farts can come out virtually odorless. An air swallower is not just blowing smoke at the skeptics when he proclaims: "Mine don't stink." He might just be a bona fide, truth-telling air swallower.

Fecal Motility Misery

Motility issues involve stools, and not the three-legged kind. Motility issues encompass a most disturbing inability to move poop loads appropriately through the colon. Such problems can result in mental anguish, critical health issues, and some very potent flatulence. People who can't move their poop are likely in the most serious category of gas passers as compared to the air swallowers or those who are chowing on too much flatulence-causing chow.

Perhaps the most important and the most common of GI disorders associated with flatulence is the irritable bowel syndrome, or IBS, as it is better known. This disease is defined by recurrent abdominal pain occurring at least once a week. Associated symptoms related to this disease include a change in frequency of bowel movements or a change in the appearances of the bowel movement. The poop production has taken on an unusual coloration or a texture that can give one pause or actually be downright frightening.

The IBS problem affects 10 to 15 percent of the population at any given time. The symptoms range from a mild nuisance to extreme discomfort to debilitating pain. Note the association of the abdominal pain with a change in bowel habits. Although not part of the specific criteria for diagnosis, abdominal bloating, and an accompanying abdominal gas, are present in almost all of the patients suffering from IBS or motility issues. From the stink standpoint, the abdominal gas output will often trump anything released by air swallowers or even those who gorge on those rascal cruciferous vegetables or their favorite red meat.

Just how intestinal gas impacts the symptoms of IBS is still an area of ongoing medical research. Some studies have shown an increase in intestinal gas in patients who experience bloating and pain, while others show the amount of gas in those with symptoms is no different than in healthy control subjects. Make no mistake, though, it can be said with some confidence that extreme constipation and motility issues do result in intestinal gas. Formal studies or anecdotal nasal notations can make that case.

The presumed mechanism of pain is thought to be a heightened sensitivity of the intestines to any intestinal gas or irritation in patients with IBS. So despite a normal amount of intestinal gas, patients with IBS may notice the symptoms of abdominal bloating and distention due to a more sensitive GI tract. The reasons behind this phenomenon are not precisely known and are still under study. It may involve a complex interaction between the nerves and muscles of the intestinal tract and the particular areas of the brain that sense pain.[7] Stay tuned.

Though IBS is not simply a gas problem, the body's ability to handle intestinal gas is certainly part of the symptom complex in IBS. In these medical patients, there are the usual suspects in determining the amount of GI gas. This includes the factors mentioned previously, including a flatulence-causing diet and air swallowing. In addition, other factors affecting increasing GI gas content include overgrowth of the bacteria that cause gas from fermentation. This goes by the acronym SIBO, which stands for small intestinal bacterial overgrowth.

Normally the bacteria in our GI system are distributed in increasing concentrations from the stomach to the small intestine to the large intestine (colon). If there are factors that disrupt this distribution and there are "too many" bacteria in the small intestine, then these bacteria can produce excess gas. Ongoing research suggests that some of these bacteria produce more of the "bad" smelly gases such as hydrogen, methane, or hydrogen sulfide.

Excess hydrogen has been associated with motility problems of the GI tract. This causes some people to have a form of IBS with loose stools of the diarrhea variety. On the other hand, an excess of methane production can lead to just the opposite, that is, IBS with predominantly rocky, concrete stools. The hard stool situation is all about constipation. Whether it's hard, lumpy poops or a chronic case of the runs, keep in mind the underlying problem of abdominal bloating and discomfort is in keeping with the diagnosis of IBS.[8]

Besides the issue of too many bacteria in the wrong place at the wrong time, there is also the issue of too many of the "bad" bacteria—read, bad gas producers—which make up a person's GI microbiome. This is a condition termed "dysbiosis" and represents a literal disruption of the normal microbiome homeostasis. As Lady Gaga might remind us, too many bad bacteria can result in a bad romance.

Among the causes of dysbiosis are illness or disease, certain medications such as antibiotics, and alcohol abuse.[9]

Good News for Farters

If there is any good news on the motility front, it's that the GI microbiome does try very hard to correct to its normal configuration once the cause of the dysbiosis has been resolved or simply disappears. Unfortunately, there is that rare person who is left with a persistent case of GI problems or irritable bowel syndrome symptoms. As an example, there are patients who have developed IBS following a severe case of infectious gastroenteritis, better known as post-infectious irritable bowel syndrome (PIIBS).[10] Everyone hates when that happens.

Almost all people with IBS experience symptomatic "flares." These can be brought on by something as simple as an imprudent evening of devouring hot wings. Another factor, which is almost universal in causing flares, is stress. And it doesn't always have to be bad stress. An upcoming wedding can trigger an onslaught of symptoms. A bride with stress-induced diarrhea may require intravenous fluids to get through a ceremony without fainting. Imagine one bridesmaid for the wedding gown train and one for the intravenous bag.

Researchers have devoted significant time, money, and publications to addressing the stress component of IBS ill effects. Studies on stress reveal that the central nervous system plays a role in IBS symptoms. Stress prompts an increase in hormonal responses that cause various effects on the body—think "flight or fight." Studies show people reporting increased anxiety and stress suffer severe IBS symptoms. Obviously, it is not possible to eliminate stress in our lives, good or bad. So what to do? Any good news? What can provide relief?

- Cognitive Behavioral Therapy (CBT). This involves diet and medical therapy. Good effects can be long lasting. CBT includes counseling, relaxation strategies, problem-solving skills, and cognitive restructuring. Basically, a person is taught to reshape the stress event, to learn to lessen its effects on the body, and to cope with effects that persist. Think of this as colon counseling.
- Hypnotherapy. Although sometimes dismissed as a "parlor trick," hypnosis can work. Hypnotherapy can address IBS symptoms and improve mood and confidence levels. This type of hypnosis is focused on the gastrointestinal tract. Under deep hypnosis, an intense meditation of sorts, one can "relax" the colon so that it is no longer prone to bloating or spasm.
- Acupuncture. Most of us are familiar with the practice of inserting needles of various sizes into specific areas of the skin to elicit a beneficial effect for medical problems. Although there is controversy on its effectiveness, acupuncture has reportedly addressed symptoms of IBS. Its goal is to "desensitize" the colon to various stimuli. This alternative method of treatment is not as well established as CBT or hypnotherapy. Like the other alternative treatments noted here, there are no real side effects—except for the discomfort of getting stuck with needles.[11]

Lest we be accused of motility issues, it's time to move on from this handy-dandy summary of categories of gas passers and their health care needs. This exploration may have been too nuts and bolts, too far into the weeds, too entangled in details and complexities for some readers. Nevertheless, any scholarly treatment of flatulence must devote a little space and time to get "down and dirty" about the causes of excess gas. So, proud fart-producer—know thyself. Embarrassed fart-producer—know thyself. Fart-producer in search of a cure—know thyself.

The facts are that everyone has intestinal gas, and everyone farts. The number and type of farts (see Chapter 3) varies from one individual to another, depending on the overall health of each person, their specific GI microbiome, and especially their diet. Hot wings or jalapeños, anyone? Those with excess or symptomatic intestinal gas may have nothing more than an increase in gas in their system due to unsettling diet or lifestyle changes.

However, if there are agonizing symptoms of discomfort or bloating, especially if these occur frequently, then it is necessary to have these symptoms checked out by a health-care professional. Specific medical conditions can be tied to excess gas and explosive flatulence. Fortunately, the majority of startling gassy conditions can be treated by dietary changes and medical or behavioral therapies. Be assured that, most of the time, excess gas is simply excess gas. And this, too, shall pass.

Consider also that there are aberrant individuals who are not interested in addressing intestinal gas issues. They thrive on the ability to release obnoxious flatulence and make themselves a public nuisance. They may, indeed, want to find ways to increase their fart production. These individuals are not just found acting in the many movies that use scenes of flatulence to entertain or gross out audiences. These people exist in real life. Do they have a psychiatric problem? Are they anti-social to the point of having a personality disorder? Is it all about toxic masculinity—just a guy thing? Is there any reason to give them a pass?

CHAPTER 5

Briefly Explained

Farts in Literature

American college students who become English majors, and who then enroll in survey courses of English literature, are often surprised that the King's English includes plenty of fiery flatulence content created by classic literary geniuses. Why the surprise? Because even though everybody farts, the mere mention of intestinal gas is considered grotesque and taboo. Those who insist that breaking wind has no place in literature or high culture are sometimes shocked to find it is an intrinsic part of the English language. In fact, the very expression "breaking wind" has existed in the United Kingdom for centuries. That common terminology presumably developed from the definition of break—meaning to start unexpectedly—and the definition of wind—meaning a flow of moving air.[1]

In medieval times, the jokers of the kingdom were practiced in the art of farting on cue and eliciting laughter among both the princely and the commoners. *The Atlantic* online magazine feature *The Daily Dish* reported in July 2007 that farts have made up a kind of language for centuries.[2] And even in medieval times, talk of farts inspired anxiety and disgust but also humor. Even in the Middle Ages, people wrestled with the notion of talking about farts because they represented a constant reminder of the undesirable behavior of the body. Flatulence provides an unavoidable awareness that the body has a mind of its own and there is nothing much you can do to change its mind. If it's going to yield to the urgency of releasing gas, well, what are you going to do about it?

In the study of English literature, Geoffrey Chaucer is often credited as the first major writer to yield to an apparently overwhelming temptation to include the cutting of the cheese as an important part of a sprawling narrative poem. Chaucer began writing his *Canterbury Tales* in 1383 when he was about 43 years old. He was several hundred years ahead of his time. English majors in American colleges learn that he employed a literary genre in his writing known as the "fabliau." Often attributed to the

French, the fabliau usually involves lower class characters who act in outrageous and even obscene ways.[3]

One of the most well-known uses of flatulence in early English literature occurs in Chaucer's *Canterbury Tales*. In the poetic episode known as "The Miller's Tale," two suitors named Nicholas and Absolon are competing for the same married woman. Nicholas, who has made his way into her bed, plots with her to humiliate his rival. When Absolon comes to her window on a dark night begging for a kiss, she presents instead her bare backside to his lips. Angered at the trick, Absolon returns later with a red-hot implement, calling for another kiss. Nicholas now brings forth his rear to release a mighty fart in Absolon's face, nearly overcoming him.

In the exact Olde English, Chaucer writes: "This Nicholas anoon leet flee a fart / As greet as it hadde been a thunder dent." Chaucer declares that this insult left Absalom both mentally and physically injured with eyes watering and throat parched: "As he were wood for wo he gan to crye / Help! Water! Water! Help, for Goddes herte." Absolon doesn't get the girl—but he does manage a well-aimed thrust of the red-hot poker. The exact consistency of the fart delivered by Nicholas upon Absolon remains unknown—perhaps a meat fart but clearly not a silent or squeaky specimen.

Approximately 200 years hence, the prolific bard of Avon, William Shakespeare, followed the bawdy example of his predecessor, Chaucer, with his own literary use of flatulence. No scholar or critic can make a solid argument for the prohibition of farts in literature when Shakespeare himself injected flatulence into his prose. Shakespeare is almost unanimously regarded as the greatest writer in the English language. His works consist of three long narrative poems, some 154 sonnets, and 39 of the greatest plays ever written. His plays are performed more often than those of any other playwright in the world. Four hundred years after his death, his stage plays continue to be performed, appreciated, studied, and reinterpreted.

Shakespeare's best known allusion to flatulence occurs in *The Comedy of Errors*. The play recounts the story of two sets of identical twins who were accidentally separated at birth. Shakespeare uses farce, slapstick, and more contrivances to exploit a case of mistaken identity. He employs other literary techniques to examine issues of family loyalty, personal persistence, and the role of coincidence in life. He resorts to a flatulence pun when the character Dromio declares: "A man may break a word with you, sir; and words are but wind; / Ay, and break it in your face, so he break it not behind."[4]

Shakespeare also had occasion to draw on metaphorical flatulence when he composed *Henry IV*, one of his more popular plays. Many of

Shakespeare's plays are complicated and full of difficult language. *Henry IV* is much easier to follow with its straightforward plot and simple conflict. As with *The Comedy of Errors*, Shakespeare resorts to talking about a human wind. It's a wind that can topple steeples and make moss-grown towers crumble. "Diseased nature oftentimes breaks forth / In strange eruptions; oft the teeming earth / Is with a kind of colic pinch'd and vex'd / By the imprisoning of unruly wind."

Henry Fielding came along in 1707, less than 100 years after the passing of William Shakespeare. Although not as prolific or recognized as Shakespeare, Fielding was dubbed the father of the modern English novel. His innovations on plot construction and the creation of story characters earned him that accolade. Fielding is famous for his novels *Joseph Andrews*, *The History of Tom Jones*, and *Shamela*. These books established Fielding as a practitioner of realism with his writing of bawdy, down-to-earth prose. He is credited with turning his back on the old age of chivalry and fantasy and recognizing the coarse reality of his time with the creation of a rambling, rapscallion fiction.

Fielding could not be completely candid in his writing with the overbearing English censors looking over his shoulder—just as they watched every other purveyor of prose in his time. Fielding dodged their reprobation by initiating the much-used tactic of strategically-located dashes in his wordsmithing. A fart became a f--t in the randy and rollicking ride known as *The History of Tom Jones*.[5] The ink-stained wretches, who set type for all the rowdy and realistic novels which emulated Fielding's works, must have had to keep a ready supply of lead dashes close at hand in their print shops.

About the same time that Fielding was perfecting the realistic novel, Jonathan Swift was exercising his skills in perfecting the satirical essay. Swift was an Anglo-Irish author born in Dublin in 1667, several decades before Fielding. Their literary periods, nevertheless, intersected. English majors and journalism majors savor the works of Jonathan Swift, whose biting satire has become a model for writers. Swift knew that writing in a satirical mode is a way to avoid the wrath of the prudes and the censors, while at the same time providing an effective way to make a point.

A Modest Proposal for preventing the Children of Poor People from being a Burthen to Their Parents or Country, and For making them Beneficial to the Publick constitutes Swift's most famous satire. In this outrageous essay, Swift proposed that the impoverished Irish might address their financial troubles by selling their children as meals for the rich. Initially, Swift appears to be drawing a sympathetic description of the plight of the impoverished in Ireland. It's shocking when he turns from this seeming heartfelt portrait and contends that "a young healthy child well nursed, is, at a year old, a most delicious nourishing and wholesome food, whether stewed, roasted, baked, or boiled; and I make no doubt that it will equally serve in a fricassee or a ragout."

Perhaps just as shocking to polite society as his modest dining proposal was Swift's impudent literary concoction titled *The Benefit of Farting Explain'd*. He penned this unique exploration into the "fundament-all cause of the distempers" under the pseudonym Professor Bum-bast of the University of Craccow with its translation for the express use of Lady Damp-Fart of Her-fart-shire, thanks to the efforts of Obadiah Fizzle, and dedicated to the Lady of Dis-stink-tion with notes by Nicholas Nincom-poop, Esq., 1722.[6]

Swift maintained that a belch is nothing but a fart half digested. And just as a gut-wrenching and bothersome belch should in no way be suppressed, neither should farts be stifled. If farts are choked back and foolishly bottled up, then erratic and outlandish behavior will most certainly result. Swift declared: "The frequent fits of Laughing and Crying, without any sensible cause (Symptoms common to such as are troubled with the Vapours), are plainly accountable from this Suppression; for the Windy Vapour getting into the Muscles that assist in laughing, inflates them, and occasions their laughing; but if this vapour, when raised to the Head, is there condensed by a cold melancholy constitution, it distills through the Eyes in the form of Tears."

Swift not only engaged in intriguing pseudo-science when describing the impact of captive intestinal gas on the average human being, but he also was one of the first writers to experiment with classifying farts. He offered details on several varieties of liberated farts that left little to the imagination. Among the species of flatulence that he described are "the sonorous and full-toned or rousing fart," "the double fart," "the soft fizzing fart," "the wet fart," and "the sullen wind-bound fart."[7] Up until this work was published, Swift's categorization was unrivaled.

In his time, Swift was in a class all by himself with his postulations on the sizes, sounds, and social impacts of flatus. Other famous English writers who have occasionally brought the essence of farting into their works, and their literary discourse, include D.H. Lawrence and James Joyce. These authors did not obsess over flatulence or use the same sardonic style as Swift, but they did find farting to be a part of life that merits curious attention. Lawrence's allusions to farts were removed by his judicious editors. Joyce's writing also ran afoul with his editors and the censors. His writing was much more guttural than Lawrence's and at times capitalized on vulgarity.

The personal correspondence of Joyce provides the clearest evidence of his fascination with flatulence, especially when the gassy phenomena becomes an integral part of sex play. In his love letters to Nora Barnacle when the lovers were in their 20s, Joyce described his joy of partaking in sex with her when she "had an arse full of farts. He described the farts as big fat fellows, long windy ones, quick little merry cracks and a lot of tiny little naughty farties." The ecstatic Joyce observed, "I think I would know Nora's fart anywhere. I think I could pick hers out in a roomful of farting women. It is a rather girlish noise not like the wet windy fart which I imagine fat wives have. It is sudden and dry and dirty like what a bold girl would let off in fun in a school dormitory at night. I hope Nora will let off no end of her farts in my face so that I may know their smell also."[8]

American Literary Flatulence

Early American literature often imitated the conceits and classicism of British literature. American writers were self-conscious about competing and equaling the quality and quantity of the mother country's literary output. It didn't help matters that after the colony broke with the empire, the English smirked, snickered, and sneered at anything coming out of the pens of the backwoods bumpkins they left behind. The Brits had an obvious advantage since English literature emerged much earlier than American literature. American literature's history dates back to the seventeenth century, whereas English literature emerged in the tenth century. English style and content naturally appeared to be richer, deeper, and more thoughtful.[9]

It did not take long, however, for American writers to establish their own literary tradition, which came to be considered simpler, more accessible, less stuffy, less inhibited. Two respected American writers who tackled the subject of flatulence and pulled it off exceedingly well are Benjamin Franklin in 1781 and Mark Twain less than a century later. The British influence is obvious in their respective pieces. Indeed, the writing could be called Swiftian. Twain's satire on flatulence actually takes a major swipe at British morals, pretensions, and mannerisms.

Franklin's writing on flatulence has been collected in a popular essay titled "Fart Proudly," and like Jonathan Swift, he argues that farts should not be restrained. He insists that such reticence to sully the atmosphere is both unnatural and unhealthy. He lists a number of maladies that can result from holding in your air. What's more, Franklin argues that releasing flatulence would not even be an issue were it not for the odiously offensive smell that often accompanies the discharging of wind from the buttocks. Franklin suggests it would be no more controversial than blowing your nose, if only for the olfactory nuisance.[10]

Always the inventor, Franklin expresses his hope that a cure will be found for the nasty odor that can accompany both the noisy variety, and the silent types, when it comes to farts:

> My Prize Question therefore should be: To discover some Drug, wholesome and not disagreeable, to be mixed with our common food, or sauces, that shall render the natural discharges of Wind from our Bodies, not only inoffensive, but agreeable as Perfumes.
>
> For the Encouragement of this Enquiry (from the immortal Honour to be reasonably expected by the Inventor) let it be considered of how small importance to Mankind, or to how small a Part of Mankind have been useful those Discoveries in Science that have heretofore made Philosophers famous. Are there twenty men in Europe at this day the happier, or even the easier for any knowledge they have pick'd out of Aristotle? What Comfort can the Vortices of Descartes give to a Man who has Whirlwinds in his Bowels!
>
> And surely such a liberty of *ex-pressing* one's *Scent-iments*, and *pleasing one another*, is of infinitely more importance to human happiness than that liberty of the *Press*, or of *abusing one another*, which the English are so ready to fight and die for."

Franklin's satirical letter of "Scent-iments" to the Royal Academy of Brussels in 1781 was never sent but was shared with his friends and later published in *Curious and Facetious Letters of Benjamin Franklin, Hitherto Unpublished, 1898.*[11]

The American writer Samuel Clemens, aka Mark Twain, was no fan or friend of royalty or empire. Twain hated all the accoutrements of monarchy and undemocratic rule. His treatise on farting in the British royal court consists of a conversation in which a fart was rudely released in the presence of the queen. No one seemed willing to take responsibility of the disgraceful emission and perhaps with good reason considering the possibilities for royal retribution. Upon reading the queen's horrified reaction to the exceedingly mighty and distressful stink of the broken wind, it's understandable that no one would want to take ownership.

> Ye Queene.—Verily in mine eight and sixty yeres have I not heard the fellow to this fart. Meseemeth, by ye grete sound and clamour of it, it was male; yet ye belly it did lurk behinde shoulde now fall lean and flat against ye spine of him yt hath bene delivered of so stately and so waste a bulk, where as ye guts of them yt doe quiff-splitters bear, stand comely still and rounde. Prithee let ye author confess ye offspring. Will my Lady Alice testify?
>
> Lady Alice Dilberry.—Good your grace, an' I had room for such a thunder-bust within mine ancient bowels, 'tis not in reason I coulde discharge ye same and live to thank God for yt He did choose handmaid so humble whereby to shew his power. Nay, 'tis not I yt have broughte forth this rich o'ermastering fog, this fragrant gloom, so pray you seeke ye further.
>
> Lady Margery Boothy.—It was not I, your maisty.[12]

The queen grows weary of all the denials. No one in the presence of the queen wants to claim the fart that has her so upset. She implores God's help, according to Twain. She asks the assembled whether they expect her to believe that the fart just tumbled from the heavens. She notes that the fart blew like a hurricane and not like the squeak of a mouse. She turns to Ben Johnson and he too denies that he was the author of the fart, but he concedes it was the product of a veteran fart producer and certainly not a novice.

Exasperated beyond her limits, the queen turns to Lord Bacon. Bacon protests that the fart was a great and mighty performance and could not have originated from his lean entrails. Bacon describes his abilities in the flatulence department as mediocre and insists that what was issued was a miracle of a fart. She then points to Shaxpur, who swears by the great hand of God that he is innocent. Shaxpur exclaimed that the noise and stink of the fart unleashed quaking thunder and firmament-clogging rottenness, so much so that heaven's artillery took notice and shook the globe in admiration of it. Finally, the queen asked Sir Walter Raleigh if he were the guilty party, and he owned up to the travesty.

"Most gracious maisty, 'twas I that did it, but indeed it was so poor and frail a note, compared with such as I am wont to furnish, yt in sooth I was ashamed to call the weakling mine in so august a presence," Sir Walter Raleigh conceded. "It was nothing—less than nothing, madam—I did it but to clear my nether throat; but had I come prepared, then had I delivered something worthy. Bear with me, please your grace, till I can make amends."[13]

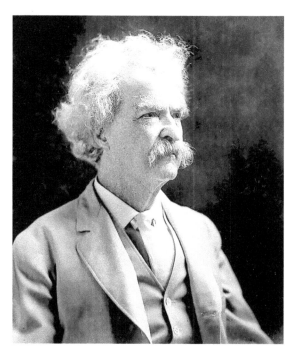

Mark Twain, who is often described as the father of American literature, never shied away from writing fantastic farting tales. In his old age, he wrote a depressing lamentation for failing sphincters that could no longer contain gas in polite company (Library of Congress).

Then Sir Walter Raleigh delivered of himself a "Godless and rock-shivering blast" that all in the queen's court and beyond were bound to close their ears to and faint upon smelling. According to Twain, there followed such a dense and foul stink that the fart which came before it seemed a poor and trifling thing—and hardly worth all the queen's consternation and interrogation.

Twain in his later years wrote some flatulence poetry that has only recently been published. His publisher cautioned him that his parody of the poem "The Rubiat of Omar Khayam" might very well disgrace him and diminish his stature with devoted readers. The poem is a lament about age with references to a "feeble stream" upon urinating. Also covered in the sorrowful complaint is unhappiness over "sphincters growing lax in their dear art," their grip diminished in whole or part.[14]

The loss of sphincter control means falling prey to a "confidence misplaced, and [we] fart in places where we should not fart." Twain's lament extends from problems passing urine to the inability to control farting to the loss of virility. Twain would probably prefer to be remembered by his fans for writing about the noise of a fart that unleashes some quaking thunder and "firmament-clogging rottenness" in a proper English setting rather than be recalled as an old codger losing sphincter control. Certainly his publisher thought so and discouraged Twain's depressing thoughts and writing on the infirmities of old age.

In the vast body of modern American literature which makes reference to farts, male characters contained therein are not shy about taking ownership of the marvelous gas that they produce. They are close kin to Mark Twain's character f Sir Walter Raleigh, who delivers a "Godless and rock-shivering blast" in the court of the queen at the time of the Tudors. In many cases, these literary allusions are all about masculinity of the most toxic kind. The ability to drop a 100-megaton methane bomb is the sign of a true alpha male. The willingness to fart in the face of a powerful enemy or a puny weakling is a sign of great masculine confidence and resolve.

The great "man's man" Ernest Hemingway also was no shrinking violet on the subject of farts in his younger years. He could undoubtedly shrivel a few violets after a long night of throwing back shots, yakking about bull fights and hunting big game, and eating the red meat of the beasts. Declared Hemingway: "Home is where the heart is, home is where the fart is, Come let us fart in the home. Still a fart may not be artless, Let us fart and artless fart in the home."[15]

Norman Mailer is another American writer whom many critics described as a "man's man" but whom others dismissed as a pretentious old fart. A Pulitzer Prize–winner like Hemingway, Mailer enjoyed rubbing readers' faces in blood and guts, cruelty and vulgarity. Mailer's *The Naked and the Dead*, a novel based on the experiences of a platoon fighting in the Philippines during World War II, provides many detailed farting scenes of men at war.

The only males who fart more than hunters of big game, or anxious troops ready for combat, are cops ready to purge the streets of low-rent evil-doers. Joseph Wambaugh's classic cop novels do not fail to take note of the noxious fumes floating through police ranks. Wambaugh's *The Choirboys* examines the inner sanctum of the Los Angeles Police Department, where neurotic young coppers harbor dark secrets of their own criminal misbehavior and sexcapades called "choir practice." The boys in the choir have backsides singing out nasty tunes which leave their superiors gasping.

Jim Dawson's *Who Cut the Cheese? A Cultural History of the Fart* documents a number of American novels with notable fart scenes. He cites E.L. Doctorow's *Ragtime* and its theme that even in the days of President William Howard Taft America was an overstuffed and farting country. He details a dog fart scene in John Irving's *Hotel New Hampshire*. He notes a "kissing the fart bubble" excerpt in a work by Philip Roth. However, Dawson eventually throws in the towel on trying to accumulate the full compendium of flatulence contained within the pages of American book writers. He confesses that such a list of sulfuric sagas could go on "ad infartnitum."[16] It's a task without end, but is it really?

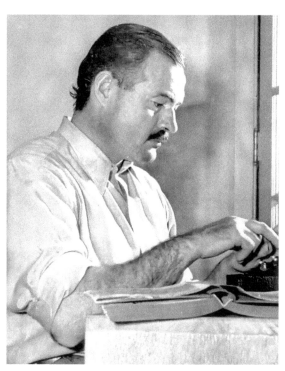

America's most manly males, writers such as Mark Twain, Ernest Hemingway, and Philip Roth, enjoyed opining on farts. Hemingway (shown here) wrote that a man's home is his castle where he should be permitted to fart both artfully and artlessly—and without censure or disapproval from anyone (Library of Congress).

Any guide or index to flatulence in the works of American authors is incomplete without mention of J.D. Salinger's classic about the hilariously alienated protagonist named Holden Caulfield. In Salinger's *The Catcher in the Rye*, narrator Caulfield tells us about a fart that nearly blows off the roof of his private school known as Pencey Prep. Caulfield is bored out of his mind listening to the sanctimonious speech of a wealthy donor in the chapel at his school. The only saving grace for the boys stuck in the chapel with the blabbering old fart comes when classmate Edgar Marsalla rips off an apparent meat fart during the intolerable speech, much to the embarrassment of the headmaster.

"The only good part of his speech was right in the middle of it. He was telling us all about what a swell guy he was, what a hotshot and all, then all of a sudden this guy sitting in the row in front of me, Edgar Marsalla, laid this terrific fart. It was a very crude thing to do, in chapel and all, but it was also quite amusing. Old Marsalla. He damn near blew the roof off," Caulfield declares in an early chapter of the Salinger novel.[17]

"Hardly anybody laughed out loud, and old Ossenburger made out like he didn't even hear it, but old Thurmer, the headmaster, was sitting right next to him on the rostrum and all, and you could tell he heard it. Boy, was he sore. He didn't say anything then, but the next night he made us have compulsory study hall in the academic building and he came up and made a speech. He said that the boy that had created the disturbance in chapel wasn't fit to go to Pencey. We tried to get old Marsalla to rip off another one, right while old Thurmer was making his speech, but he wasn't in the right mood," Caulfield laments.[18]

Edgar Marsalla's infamous fictional fart no doubt inspired many real farts to be cut at inappropriate moments in schools across the United States after the novel was published in 1951. *Catcher in the Rye* was banned by many schools, even though it was on the *New York Times* bestseller list week after week. The controversial book shaped American adolescent culture and established a unique brand of American-style youth rebellion—the kind of rebellion that has included "terrific farts being laid" in defiance of established authority.

Chaucer, Fielding, and Shakespeare all had their moments expounding on flatulence in their contributions to English literature. No one can hold a candle—nor should they try to hold a candle—to the flatulence expositions of two giants, Benjamin Franklin and Mark Twain. Nevertheless, J.D. Salinger holds a special place in the annals of American anal emission scenes and all of world literature for that matter. Salinger is the king when it comes to creating a fart that changed the world, and his book detailing Edgar Marsalla's fart has sold more than 65 million copies.

CHAPTER 6

Noise Over Children's Fart Books

A troubled youngster in the children's book *My Butt Is So Noisy* has a posterior problem. The hooting and tooting from his hind end gets him into trouble with adult authority figures as well as close relatives. He feels badly about himself in the early pages of the well-illustrated tale created by Dawn McMillan. His butt is capable of putting out such a wide range of unpleasant tones and aromas that the local press comes running to see what all the commotion is about. The press saves the day and his butt.

By the end of *My Butt Is So Noisy*, McMillan's youthful farting phenom becomes a media celebrity.[1] The news media have caught wind of his special attribute and the once-troubled youngster takes a newfound pride in himself. A chauffeur drives him around a large metropolis where he takes great enjoyment in his sonorous butt and its exceptional range of fart releases. Life is good in children's fart book world.

Once upon a time, children were to be seen—but only just barely. Certainly they were not to be heard and absolutely not to be smelled. In the 1950s and 1960s era of *Leave It to Beaver*, *Father Knows Best*, and *Ozzie and Harriet* television shows, children were the disenfranchised and subservient members of the nuclear family unit. They had no say or vote in family decision-making. They were to listen and do as they were told or face the consequences. They devoted their time to completing daily chores and earning spending money at part-time jobs, except when they were attending school and cracking the books for their homework.

Above all children were expected to behave, to be courteous and well-mannered. There was an ingrained ritual of saying "please" and "thank you" and there was never any swearing. Kids of that era were never permitted to put elbows on the table or to wear a baseball cap, frontward or backward, while sharing in the family meal. Knife and fork were held in the correct manner. Chewing was done with mouth closed. Mouth and nose were covered in the event of a cough or a sneeze. An accidental burp was followed by a red face and a very sincere "excuse me." The emission of a fart—be it an unintended squeaker or a low-volume barking spider—was simply out of the question.

All that has changed. Author McMillan's child prodigy is just one of many examples of the new age of not only letting it "all hang out" but also letting it all rip and waft. By the end of McMillan's book, the child wonder is sporting microphones, speakers, and an audio control console strapped to his musical backside. The spectacle is illustrated by artist Ross Kinnaird. The boy's noisy butt has become a cornucopia of joy, jocularity, and pride—and also a source of squealing, staccato screeching, and rolling thunder.

Parents of a new century may find McMillan's book amusing and may also be tickled to find their own children trying to emulate the exploits of the boy with the noisy butt. These modern parents also may take satisfaction in the notion that they are raising their kids in a relaxed environment where no shame is attached to doing what comes naturally. However, more traditional parents are not so pleased with this trend in literary choices for the pint-sized. The book also has been banned in some school libraries and school employees in the South have been reprimanded for reading *My Butt Is So Noisy* to kids. Undoubtedly, there are more discordant noises to come over the controversial children's books that are accused of promoting bad manners.

Some might blame the dramatic disappearance of manners and courtesy among the younger set on the making of the counter culture in the 1970s. However, that was the hippie revolution among those of college age and beyond. Young children of that time were not wearing granny glasses and sporting Afros, nor were they adopting the language of liberation or giving a middle finger to the establishment. To be sure, some aspects of the counter culture did seep down to the world of grade schoolers and kindergarteners. These youngsters would later become parents. In point of fact, though, the real insurrection of the youngest among us came in the 1990s and early 21st century with what can appropriately be termed the "Grossness Revolution."

The Grossness Revolution—characterized by a wave of flagrant atrociousness, egregiousness, outrageousness, and rankness—continues to resound and afflict us today. Some experts trace its beginnings to the unusual children's books written by Sylvia Branzei. The first book in 1992, *Grossology*, is a frank, no-holds-barred examination of gross bodily functions that previously were the province of the doctor's office. The book was an immediate hit with children, but many parents found it unappealing and purchased copies with understandable reluctance.

Slimy, Mushy, Oozy....

The book's major topics are classified under three headings: "Slimy Mushy Oozy Gross Things," which includes urine, diarrhea, vomit, acne, and blisters; "Crusty Scaly Gross Things," which includes dandruff and tooth decay; and "Stinky Smelly Gross Things," which covers bad breath, extreme halitosis, fart noises, and general flatulence.[2] The success of the initial *Grossology* book inspired Branzei to write sequels such as *Stinky Smelly Gross Things* and *Animal Grossology*. The animal stars in her 1996 book include tapeworms and dung beetles, creatures that she has classified as "Dookie Lovers."

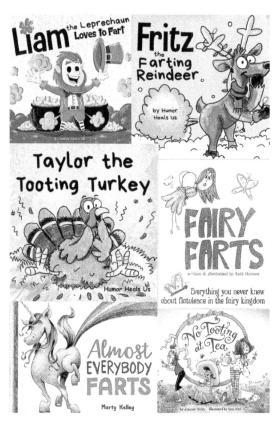

The initial dookie tracts of the Grossness Revolution inspired a torrent of flatulence literature and illustrated fart books for children. Among the titles now available for kids are *Even Fairies Fart, No Tooting at Tea, Rudy's Windy Christmas, The World's Biggest Fart, Where Is My Butt*, and *Almost Everybody Farts*. The Grossness Revolution has proven not to be some mere passing fad. It's here to stay and there's no putting the genie, or anything else, back in the bottle. Parents who yearn to make farting taboo once again are dreaming and in for a rude awakening. They're on the wrong side of history. And today's experts on childhood and adolescence simply itch to pontificate on why history is on the side of flatulence.

Holiday fart books for children are in ample supply with farting turkeys, gassy leprechauns, and rascally reindeer. Farting princesses, flatulent fairies, and fumigating unicorns also abound in today's children's literature (photograph by Ursula Ruhl).

Consultant and author Lisa Ferland argues that parents who refuse to buy their kids books about farts need to wake up and smell the coffee and whatever else might be in the air. She contends parents need to be more open-minded and acknowledge that 99 percent of kids will giggle and say yes when asked if farts are funny. Parents need to quit being prudish and uncomfortable and just join in the fun, according to Ferland. She offers five big reasons for rethinking flatulence and children in her essay "Why We Need More Kids' Books About Farts."[3]

Ferland's first fart finding is that laughing about a taboo topic such as farting can open up an honest dialogue between adult and child. She argues that having frequent conversations about minor issues like farting can pave the way for future discussions about more serious topics like reproduction, pregnancy, sexual identity, abusive behaviors, and much more. According to Ferland, if an adult has to struggle to talk about normal bodily functions, how can they be expected to handle the really tough topics as kids grow older? If adults read to youngsters about flatulence, kids will learn that they can safely talk about any problem that they might be facing in their future.

The Ferland exposition offers four more points in defense of children's fart books. She explains that the key to literacy for children is to develop their love for reading. If kids are obsessed with stories about underpants or farting, then stock up on the books that cover these subjects. It's better for kids to be reading something they like than nothing at all. Why not let teachers force the boring stuff on them? Besides, there will be plenty of time for the classics, but without a critical love for reading, they're never going to get to Shakespeare.

There is also a therapeutic benefit to children reading fart books, according to Ferland. She maintains that normalizing fart behavior can help youngsters with self-worth and body image issues. Fart books are really good for girls to read, because that can help with their tendency to hate their bodies and normal body processes. She insists it's past time for girls to stop thinking that it's grievously wrong for them to fart, and boys need to stop thinking that girls who fart are gross and fair game for bullying.

Ferland makes two more points that appear to be tailored to authors and those interested in breaking into the writing business. She suggests that reading and writing a fart book can be a humorous experience that relieves stress and tensions. She claims that authors who turn up their noses at creating fart books simply don't realize there is a hot market for high-quality flatulence works that can make kids laugh. She notes the considerable regret of highbrow book writers who cannot score even one Amazon reader review. In contrast, a book like *I Need a New Bum* has garnered hundreds of 5-star reviews. Likewise, *Walter the Farting Dog* has more than 600 5-star reviews.

One author who has found fame, fans and fun serving the needs of the children's fart book market is Jane Bexley, who has created the Toot Along Story Series and the Fart Dictionary Series. Some selections from Bexley's assorted toot tales include *Gary the Goose and His Gas on the Loose, Dad & Me Setting Farts Free, Turkey Toots Save the Day, Harvey the Heart Had Too Many Farts*, and *Monster Farts*. Bexley's Fart Dictionary Series includes *Freddie the Farting Snow Man, Larry the Farting Leprechaun,* and *Princesses Don't Fart (They Fluff)*.

Freddie the Farting Snow Man from the Fart Dictionary Series lacks a plot, but the snowman does offer a potpourri of different farts that make up the life of a snowman. The icy farts range from the Arctic Blast to the Farticle Collider. Some readers are disappointed not to find a whimsical tale within the covers of the snowman book. Other readers retort that the book is not meant to be a story with a beginning and an end and a moral. Rather, the book is a catalog of fantastic fantasy farts from the land of ice, igloos, and maybe a few Inuits.[4]

Dad & Me Setting Farts Free from Bexley's Toot Along Story Series is about a little bear who tries to be just like his papa in every way, including popping booty burns from the old bear's buttocks. Some readers contend this book is going to elicit more laughs from dads than from the small fry. Therefore, it makes a good Father's Day present for the dad who loves his flatulence as well as the dad who is still in the initial stages of learning the fine art of reading for Junior before bedtime.[5]

Fart Humor Heals Us?

The publisher of Humorhealsus Books has the widest selection of children's fart books. These include two in which the protagonists are tooting turkeys; two in which the main characters are farting leprechauns; and two in which the farting story subjects are pooting penguins. The books in the Humorhealsus series of children's fart books are very often tailored for the holidays.

Thanksgiving is the perfect time to acquire either one of the two Taylor the Turkey books. Christmas is the perfect time to consider either one of the two Fritz the Farting Reindeer books. However, if reindeer are not your thing at Christmas, then Santa's Tooting Tooshie may be the correct choice as a stocking stuffer. Santa Claus jokes that he keeps Fritz the Farting Reindeer in the back row of his sleigh team. This is a credit to the jolly old man's wit and wisdom.[6]

Some fart books seem more appropriate for the sensibilities of young girls, while others seem especially tailored for the kind of boyish sense of fart humor commonly shared by a father and his son. Two books that have lessons for young girls are *Princesses Don't Fart (They Fluff)* and *Fairy Farts: Everything You Never Knew About Flatulence in the Fairy Kingdom.* The princesses are a production of Jane Bexley, writer and illustrator. The fairies are a production of Kelli Hansen, writer and illustrator.[7]

The message of Bexley's book is that princesses do, indeed, have gas. However, a polite princess knows there is a time and a place for every kind of toot. Soft "twinkle toots" can be loosed in a dance class, and if they can be synchronized with all the other dancers, so much the better. The "fumigator" should only be launched outside and preferably in a flower garden where delightful scents of budding plants can mix in and dilute the fumigator fart. At the end of the day, a princess can safely launch a few bath bombs in the privacy of her royal bathroom.

The message of Hansen's book is that fairies do, indeed, have gas. Fairies do try to modulate the audio emissions of their farts, so that their sound is much more of a poof of air than a noisy toot. This is somewhat impractical because the author maintains that fairies' favorite food is the bean burrito. Chili cook-offs also are a popular event for fairies, so they have a particularly noisome challenge being discreet with their gas. Nevertheless, fairies are pretty good at keeping things under control and confining any stinky business to poofs.

Children's fart books for boys are not usually about quiet princess twinkle toots or barely audible fairy poofs. Boys are inclined to enjoy a book about something more substantial. Two books that have lessons for young boys are *Dad & Me Setting Farts Free* and *My Dad Loves to Toot.* The father and son farting team is a production of Jane Brexley, writer and illustrator. The proud toot-producing dad is a production of an author whose pen name is Tootin' Tom.

The message of Bexley's *Dad & Me Setting Farts Free* is that every little baby bear wants to be just like his big daddy bear in every way, and that includes emulating flatulence behavior. The two bears ride a motorcycle together, a vehicle that seems to derive some of its propulsion and lift from dad's expulsions. Reviewers say the rhyming text and colorful illustrations make the book memorable for more than just its hilarity.

The message of Tootin' Tom's *My Dad Loves to Toot* is all about the boundless love of a son for his father. Dad can do no wrong and his rather strange affection for his own flatulence both amuses and awes his son. The son relates how his dad passes gas in both his state of sleep and his waking hours. His dad toots at important business meetings. His dad toots while in line at the grocery store, much to the chagrin of women behind him. His dad toots in the evening as the family sits on the couch watching television. The son testifies that dad is his hero and some day he hopes that he will learn to play the "trouser flute" just as well.[8]

Off-Putting, Obnoxious, Outrageous

There is no question that children's fart books can be off-putting, obnoxious, outrageous, and arguably obscene. Advocates still argue that the books are important for little girls and boys in teaching life lessons. The lessons do not have much to do with manners or common courtesy or behaving in polite society. In the case of lessons imparted for girls, there does sometimes seem to be a message that while farting is inevitable, discretion can be the better part of valor. In the case of little boys, the message seems to be that farting can be a badge of honor. And, what's more, reading about farts can be fun. In fact, the overriding salvation of an obnoxious fart book for little boys is that it keeps them interested and reading.

This overriding salvation was emphasized in a story on the learning crisis of boys in American schools in a 2010 Associated Press (AP) article by Leanne Italie. The article noted that boys have lagged behind girls in reading achievement for decades. The gender gap now exists in nearly every state and has widened to mammoth proportions— as much as 10 percentage points in some states, according to the Center on Education Policy. The arti-

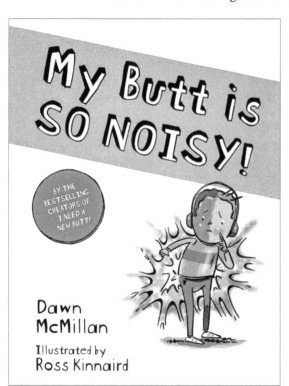

Children's books such as *My Butt Is So Noisy* and *I Need a New Butt* stir up plenty of controversy. Fart books for boys can raise the roof when brought to school. Disciplinary measures have resulted not only for students but also for offending teachers and administrators (photograph by Ursula Ruhl).

cle discusses whether fart jokes and fart books can save the reading souls of boys.

Teachers, librarians, and concerned parents interviewed for the AP article were all in agreement that the answer is a resounding yes. Butts. Farts. Underpants. Whatever gross subject gets boys to read, go for it. Amelia Yunker, a children's librarian in Farmington Hills, Michigan, recalled hosting a grossology party with slime and an armpit noise demonstration. "Just get 'em reading," she said. "Worry about what they're reading later."

A fourth grade teacher in Raleigh, North Carolina, Cathy Walker, said she also is constantly looking for ways to engage hard-to-reach boys. She stumbled on Ray Sabini's volume on flatulence, *SweetFarts*, read it for herself and knew it would be a hit: "It's a topic most teachers and parents don't openly discuss," she said. "It's a great way for boys to engage in topics that are 'taboo' and because of that, they enjoy them even more."[9]

The amazing takeaway message from the burgeoning children's fart book movement is this: Don't take farts, or books about farts, so seriously. These children's books will help you bond and connect with your kids. They will help you have rich conversations about important matters later on in life. However, parents may want to advise their children not to imitate the flatulence of story characters at school. School administrators and teachers still frown on classroom cheese-cutting. And some school board members are always looking for the next school book to ban.

CHAPTER 7

News Coverage

Law and Odor

Flatulence is a multi-media topic. Hollywood film producers, cable television companies, legacy news media, and the new social media have all found that farts can attract an audience. How they use and shape flatulence content depends on the nature of the particular medium. It's worth drawing on the observations of the late multi-media expert Marshall McLuhan to put flatulence in context.

Movies push the envelope with flatulence. When the main characters are not lighting up their gas in great balls of fire and blue flame explosions, they are weaponizing their farts to humiliate their friends and enemies. Movie characters in films usually take ownership of their noxious flatulence productions or they point fingers and try to blame innocent pets and hapless humans for their odorous indiscretions. It's all in good fun, though, because movies are all about entertainment.

Cable television provides a venue for outrageous comedy routines about flatulence. Traditional television, on the other hand, has shied away from most fart content for fear of running afoul of Federal Communications Commission (FCC) regulations. The word "fart" has been deemed as an eighth dirty word, an ugly little four-letter word that merits censorship. This is in line with the original "seven dirty words" formulated by comedian George Carlin. "Fart" is the other f-bomb that nobody wants to own virtually or otherwise on regular TV. However, when it comes to cable television, the doors have been thrown wide open for fart talk.

Cable television has provided a platform for plenty of new flatulence comedians. They cut their teeth on fart banter and comedy routines all about cutting the cheese. Cable television comes into homes by choice and is paid for by subscribers. Don't want to hear jokes about farts? Media industry regulators advise cutting the wire, axing the cable subscription, or taking the satellite dish off the roof. In any case, it's all just raunchy fun, and cable's comedy channels are all about entertainment.

The legacy media of newspapers are an entirely different matter. Newspapers are ostensibly in the business of providing information. It's all about news that you can use. Granted, newspapers will package their information pieces in a variety of ways. Over the years, the newspaper press has developed different genres, such as tabloid, yellow, and muckraking journalism. News about farts will be packaged according to the needs of each selected genre.

Media guru Marshall McLuhan told us that the medium is the message.[1] The medium of film has a very different mission than that of the printed word. The newspapers displayed in vending boxes have a very different mission than that of the television screen delivering images via cable. The wired world is different than the world of ink on paper, as McLuhan insisted on shaping his own message for media scholars.

McLuhan told us that news media information in newspapers is generally "hot" and serious. Newspaper content is less about entertainment and more about informing you about serious issues. In the case of flatulence, the news is all about learning the ins and outs of the various "sides" on cutting the cheese—and perhaps even urging you to take a stand. Where do you stand on flatulence expression? What is your opinion on gas expulsions in the public sphere? Newspaper opinion pages and editorials may advise you regarding what your stance should be on farting content in school books and television entertainment.

Newspaper opinions on flatulence emissions harken back to the classic song by Matron "Mama" Morton and Velma Kelly in the musical *Chicago*. The two actresses nostalgically lament that society no longer values kindness, manners, and restraining unwanted fumes. Everyone is on the make and acts like a snake in the grass. Good breeding is a thing of the past. "Please" and "thank you" are forgotten niceties. Manners are in short supply. Mama Morton and Velma bemoan the fact that now "no one even says 'oops' when they're passing their gas. Whatever happened to class?"[2]

"Whatever happened to fair dealing, and pure ethics, and nice manners?" moan the jailhouse ladies in *Chicago*. The news media sing out of that same playbook with their opinion pieces. Why are our so-called leaders telling fake stories and lies, belittling others, and behaving like uncouth children? Why are social media and the Internet just plain crude? These questions are being asked by the secular press as well as by the religious media and weekly newspapers of different denominations.

The religious press looks to the basic precept of Jesus Christ for guidance with his words in Matthew 7:12—"Do unto others as you would have them do unto you." That means you don't fart in the presence of others, lest ye be farted upon. Unrestrained flatulence is a sure sign of selfishness, self-absorption, incivility, and a vulgarity that borders on sinfulness.

What's more, these social infractions engender hostility in the workplace and malevolence directed at school and civil officials. Insults are even hurled at shop clerks and flight attendants.

The secular press relies less on religious doctrine and more upon the imperatives of the social contract when it opines on farting. That means we don't fart in the presence of others, because we are all on this planet together. The planet is growing smaller, so burping and farting, picking and licking, rolling and flicking make living in more crowded spaces simply intolerable. To avoid nastiness and violence, we must make the effort to adhere to the collective good and respect some obvious physical and psychic boundaries.

So who is to blame for all the rudeness and displays of flatulence? Editorials take aim at any number of bad actors. Among the culprits are the misbehavior of religious authorities and the decline of religion. Craven politicians also take the blame for aping the vulgarities of their crude followers rather than leading by uplifting example. The media industry itself takes it on the chin for providing a steady stream of cringeworthy entertainment fare. Psychologists get a share of the blame for excusing infantile behavior because of anxiety in a time of pandemic, social upheaval, and economic dislocation.

Then there is the whole "grossology phenomenon." Educators are writing children's books advising them that social niceties can take a back seat to natural bodily functions. Go ahead and fart, Jacky and Tommy. It's okay to act out with our bodily effluvia—peeing, pooping, belching, and farting—because, after all, that is what nature intended. Close behind the grossologists are all the licentious free thinkers and their situation ethics and moral relativity. The old authorities on social norms and appropriate behavior must yield to the needs and demands for individual freedom—to fart.

Tabloid, Yellow, and Mucky

In contrast to the anger and the finger-pointing in news editorials on flatulence in media outlets, tabloid journalism has prospered by actually exploiting the underside—and backside—of human experience for sensationalism. Outrageous scandals, disgusting deviancy, high crimes, and pathetic misdemeanors involving low-life farting—all have hit the front pages of the tabloid press. A catalog of top tabloid newspaper accounts on flatulence includes sordid tales involving political figures, petty criminals, old farts with out-of-control gas problems, and truly aberrant human behavior in public settings.

Political junkies will never forget tabloid news accounts of U.S. Congressman Eric Swalwell allegedly breaking wind during a live TV interview at the time of the Trump impeachment. True crime buffs relish reading stories of thieves hiding from police and having their covers blown by their own noisy flatulence. Fans of muckraking eagerly read and share stories about livestock flatulence and how the agriculture industry is doing squat to stop dangerous climate change caused by farting cows. As the atmosphere heats up, expect more muckraking and yellow journalism exposing a careless farm industry letting cattle add their methane to the atmosphere.

Stories also abound in the tabloid press about farting crooks and their propensity for getting in trouble with the law. Sometimes even law enforcement gets in trouble for farting. Weird and outrageous tabloid journalism originated in Britain but was exported to the United States after World War I. Today's tabloids in the United States are most often found in supermarket checkout lanes or in the vending boxes of the Big Apple that carry the *New York Post* or the *New York Daily News*. In Britain, the most famous tabloids have included *The Sun, The Daily Mirror,* and the *Daily Mail*.

Some of the most unusual fart incident stories have come from the British tabloids over the years and then inspired similar stories in the U.S. press. A London *Daily Mail* story in 2001 detailed a drug raid in which an officer farted loudly during the law enforcement actions. The family subjected to the fart lodged a complaint and Scotland Yard investigated. The *Daily Mail* then printed a department incident report: "An allegation has been received from a person in the house that one of the male officers

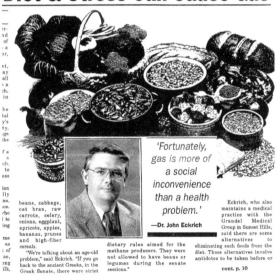

Diet & Stress Can Cause Gas

'Fortunately, gas is more of a social inconvenience than a health problem.'
—Dr. John Eckrich

beans, cabbage, oat bran, raw carrots, celery, onions, eggplant, apricots, apples, bananas, prunes and high-fiber cereals.

"We're talking about an age-old problem," said Eckrich. "If you go back to the ancient Greeks, in the Greek Senate, there were strict

dietary rules aimed for the methane producers. They were not allowed to have beans or legumes during the senate sessions."

Eckrich, who also maintains a medical practice with the Grandel Medical Group in Sunset Hills, said there are some alternatives to eliminating such foods from the diet. Those alternatives involve antidotes to be taken before or

cont. p. 10

Newspaper stories such as this 1992 article about holiday diet and flatulence problems are relatively rare. However, the New York tabloid press has run a number of stories about crooks tracked down and apprehended because of their telltale gas passing (courtesy *Webster-Kirkwood Times*).

broke wind and did not apologize to the family for his action … the complainant felt it was rude and unprofessional."[3]

Another story from Aberdeen, Scotland, related how a suspect for drug offenses farted aggressively at approaching police and taunted them, saying, "How do you like that?" Officers apprehended him after "they got wind that something was amiss when they saw him at the side of the road following a crash." The judge in the case did not let his aggressive farting pass, and the gassy insult to the police was weighed heavily in his sentencing.[4]

A more recent story from the East Midlands of Britain in 2020 told of a crime suspect who hid in a heavily wooded area near Harworth, Nottinghamshire. His location remained a mystery until officers got close and heard the unmistakable sound of breaking wind. Another suspect was arrested after he was found hiding behind a nearby house. The story was headlined "A Wanted Man Who Hid in Bushes Blew His Cover When He Farted." A pursuing officer was quoted, "I was almost out of wind running but luckily the suspect still had some."[5]

American tabloids also will never take a pass on a good gas-passing story. They find instruction in the British tabloid press. In 1994, the *Daily News* in New York reported on a "career criminal" who was burglarizing a home in Fire Island, New York. Residents were startled and went downstairs to investigate unusual noises. The burglar hid in the closet and probably would have escaped notice, but he was unable to restrain his gas. A resident opened the closet door upon hearing the motorboat sound of the staccato escaping flatulence. The burglar was restrained until police could arrive and take control of the crime scene.[6]

Another alarming gas-passing story out of Liberty, Missouri, received attention not only in news outlets in the Midwest. The story also wafted its way across the Atlantic to the British tabloids. According to the *Kansas City Star*, police in the Kansas City suburb were searching in vain for a man wanted for possession of a controlled substance. He was trying to evade police, but law enforcement detected where he was hiding when he let out a loud blast. The Clay County Sheriff's Department congratulated the Liberty police with a Facebook post: "We've got to give props to Liberty PD for using their senses to sniff him out."[7]

And then there's that story in the American news media about the live television fart pinned on U.S. Representative Eric Swalwell, D–California. The *Washington Examiner* blew a hole in that story when it reported in November 2019 that the FCC had been urged to investigate Swalwell's "disgusting, vulgar display" that "has no place on live television." The *Examiner* quipped that the FCC Chairman Ajit Pai cut a cheesy statement in reply: "I hate to cause a stink, but we have to decline the invitation; any

FCC investigation would abruptly run out of gas given that this alleged emission occurred on a cable news network—the relevant rules apply only to broadcast television," Pai said.[8]

The fart noise, which sounded like a chair scraping across the floor, could be heard as Swalwell spoke with MSNBC host Chris Matthews. The clip immediately went viral, and the Twitter world assumed it was Swalwell who dealt it. Donald Trump, Jr., sarcastically claimed it was the "most intelligible thing to come out of Swalwell in years. #fartgate." The hashtags #fartgate and #shartgate subsequently exploded on social media.

Swalwell took pains to deny that he broke wind live on cable, while some observers then suggested that Matthews was the probable cause of the flatulence disturbance. MSNBC's *Hardball* subsequently tweeted that the noise heard by viewers was actually a mug scraping across the desk in their studio. The cable network noted: "Sorry to disappoint the conspiracy theorists—it was a *Hardball* mug scraping across the desk. Get yours today and let's get back to the news!"[9]

Flatulence and Media Regulation

Newspapers and news media outlets occasionally rise above the scolding editorial opinions and sensational tabloid coverage of flatulence phenomena. These exceptions occur when journalists write serious, in-depth analysis pieces on free expression issues and flatulence. Because this kind of writing involves complex First Amendment law, it gets complicated. It also can get very political as there are some major philosophical differences among social conservatives, liberals, and libertarians as to what is appropriate journalism and protected expression—even in the rather benign realm of flatulence.

When judges on the U.S. Supreme Court and members of the Federal Communications Commission lean toward a social conservative philosophy, they are sometimes tempted to put the lid on flatulence. After all, flatulence is utterly without redeeming social values. It's disgusting speech that does not merit protection. However, the news and entertainment media generally support the free flow of flatulence information. They will protest attempts by judges and commissioners to quash or curtail content involving flatulence.

When judges and commission members lean toward a liberal philosophy or libertarian absolutist position on the First Amendment, they will oppose the heavy hand of censorship. The media then find that they have friends in high places supporting their publishing or airing questionable flatulence content. The judicial quandary for all the various parties involved is whether extreme flatulence material constitutes profane, obscene, or indecent content.

In recent years, courts and regulatory agencies have tried to draw distinctions on what constitutes obscene content, indecent content, and profane content. *Obscene content* is not covered by rights of free expression and the protection of the First Amendment. For content to be ruled obscene, it must meet the three-pronged test established by rulings of the Supreme Court: It must appeal to an average person's prurient interest; depict or describe sexual conduct in a "patently offensive" manner; and, taken as a whole, be devoid of any serious literary, artistic, political, or scientific value.

Indecent content depicts sexual or excretory organs or such activities in a way that is patently offensive but does not meet the three-prong test for obscenity. Broadcast media has sometimes regulated indecent content by prohibiting it during hours when children would be awake and have access to it. Indecent material is therefore restricted from airing on television and radio between the hours of 6 a.m. and 10 p.m. *Profane content* includes "grossly offensive" language that is considered a public nuisance.

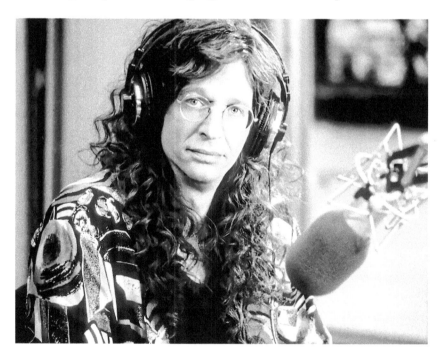

Self-described fartman Howard Stern has found plenty of media coverage in the entertainment and business pages of American newspapers. His gassy brand of humor has established an unrivaled reputation as a top-grossing radio shock jock (Paramount Pictures/Photofest).

So where does flatulence content fall among these three categories? It's all in the eyes and ears of the beholder. When shock jocks on the radio start talking about vaginal farts and flatulence during sex, that is content which can easily wander into the sphere of what is obscene. On the other hand, if the radio deejays are simply talking about different varieties of fart noises and airing some of these noises, the content could be indecent but not obscene from a legal standpoint. Violations in these content areas can result in monetary fines placed on broadcast station owners or even forfeiture of a federal broadcast license.

Although the general public will have widely varying opinions on what kind of flatulence content is criminally obscene and what is simply indecent, court judges are expected to be much more adept at drawing the lines. However, even U.S. Supreme Court judges can disagree with each other and have difficulty making distinctions over obscenity, indecency, or a simple public nuisance. As Supreme Court Justice Potter Stewart said in 1964: "I shall not today attempt further to define the kinds of material I understand to be embraced within that shorthand description [obscenity], and perhaps I could never succeed in intelligibly doing so. But I know it when I see it...."[10]

Do high court justices, judges, and commissioners really know it when they see it? *Rolling Stone* and other magazines have published articles slamming judges and regulatory agencies for their imprecision and confusion on obscenity. In 2004, *Rolling Stone* painted a chaotic picture of recent regulatory efforts, noting the FCC had fined broadcasters more than $1.5 million, busted NBC for U2 singer Bono's accidental use of the f-bomb on its air, and ruled that fart sounds are against the law. "It's absurd," Lou Reed of the Velvet Underground told *Rolling Stone*. "It's like being censored by a squirrel. It's beneath me, it's beneath all these artists. It's done by people who are very pious and stupid."[11]

Pious and stupid or not, judges and courts can cause a lot of headaches for artists and media companies trying to parse the difference between obscenity and lesser offenses. The FCC has further muddied the picture by deciding that the indecency and profanity prohibitions apply to "conventional broadcast services" but not to subscription media such as cable television, satellite, and Internet services. Legacy broadcast media are crying "unfair" because they are losing audience to the new media that can offer edgier material without penalty and achieving high ratings.

In 2008, journalist Matthew Lasar wrote that Clear Channel Communications was among the legacy broadcasters tired of being fined for "edgy" content. Clear Channel also had lost patience seeing its edgy talent move to SiriusXM satellite radio. On-air talent who made the move to satellite radio could subsequently be indecent and profane without penalty.[12]

"In referring to being fined for 'edgy' content, Clear Channel probably means the voice of Howard Stern, now broadcasting on channels 100 and 101 of Sirius satellite radio," Lasar wrote. "In 2004 the FCC slapped six Clear Channel stations with almost half-a-million dollars in fines for airing a program in which Stern and his guests discussed anal and oral sex while sounds that resembled farting aired in the background. The agency also took exception to Stern's praise of an imaginary personal hygiene product identified as 'Sphincterine'; flatulence could also be heard during this segment."[13]

Two months later, Clear Channel settled with the FCC for the Stern programs and other radio fare that the agency identified as indecent. Clear Channel agreed to pay the government $1.75 million and set up a company-wide plan for preventing indecent broadcasting on its licenses. The broadcaster also removed Howard Stern from its stations. In October 2004, Stern announced that he would leave terrestrial radio entirely and move to Sirius. "It's time to go," Stern told his listeners. "I believe more in satellite than I do in radio."[14]

CHAPTER 8

Breaking Bad

Entertainment Media

It's impossible to talk about flatulence in entertainment without giving the master "flatulist" of all time his due. That would be the French entertainer Le Pétomane whose miraculous control of his stomach muscles allowed him to perform farting feats known to few mortal men. His stage name, Le Pétomane, is a combination of the French word "to fart" and the word for "maniac." In other words, "fart maniac." The man who entertained tens of thousands during his 88-year lifetime that began in 1857 literally was named the "fart maniac."

Le Pétomane's real name was Joseph Pujol. His flatulence abilities often were mistakenly attributed to a consumption of beans and high-fiber foods that resulted in extreme intestinal gas. Gastroenterologists are now able to explain that Pujol's abilities were because he was an air swallower, not because he had an unusual diet or motility problems. He was, however, an unusual air swallower because he did not take in huge amounts of air through the mouth but through the entrance of his back end. He exercised his ability to inhale air into his rectum and then modulated the release of that air with his agile anal sphincter muscles.

The name Le Pétomane was popularized in the United States with the publication of the book by the same name through Los Angeles–based publisher Sherbourne Press. Jean Nohain and F. Caradec's 1967 book *Le Pétomane* was a sensation among American readers. The publicity generated on the radio-television promotional circuit had the book flying off the store shelves for years. In 1993, the book was picked up by Dorset Press of Barnes & Noble and continued to fascinate American readers.

The Sherbourne Press edition of *Le Pétomane* notes that here was a strangely talented man who "shook and shattered the Moulin Rouge— and shocked even the broad-minded Parisians."[1] The authors recounted the scenes of his performances in the great theater as simply delirious and impossible to describe. His audiences began to shout, their faces turned apoplectic, their cheeks were covered with streams of tears. Their visages reflected amusement and amazement.

"Someone would be stricken with a crazy laugh. In a moment people would be howling and staggering with laughter," observed Nohain and Caradec, who then noted that things could turn serious. "Some would stand paralyzed, tears pouring down their cheeks.... Ladies would begin to suffocate in their tight corsets, and for this reason there were always a number of white-coated nurses in attendance."[2]

So what happened at a Le Pétomane stage act to merit such a madcap response? Le Pétomane would come on stage, dressed smartly in dark coat, red breeches, white stockings, and patent leather shoes. There was no nudity in his show because he could perform his act through the fabric of his trousers. His act could include a series of flatulence expulsions, which he would describe as a bride on her wedding night, or as a dressmaker tearing yards of material, or as a large cannon discharging during war time. He might conclude his act by breaking a blast of wind to blow out a candle with his appropriately aimed buttocks more than a foot away.

Sometimes Le Pétomane would give private performances to the very wealthy to provide more insight into his abilities. He would appear in a bathing costume with a great opening cut in the back which allowed for a rubber hose. His hose demonstrations would include cigarette and flute performances. The finale might have Le Pétomane lowering himself into a basin of water and pumping the liquid into himself and then expelling it in a virtual fire brigade stream under enormous pressure.

Le Pétomane discovered his gift when as a little boy he went to the beach with his family. He placed his head under water and, holding his breath, he was astonished to find the icy cold water entering his stomach through his anus. When he ran up on the beach he was frightened to see the water pouring out of him. His mother took him to the doctor, who dismissed the occurrence as "nothing." However, as a young adult, Joseph Pujol began experimenting with his unique talent and his friends began to praise his abilities as astonishing.

Pujol realized that he could take in as much water as he wished and project a water spout. He also could replace water with air. After sucking in the air, Pujol could release it in varying amounts and create a catalog of noisy farts with a minimum of sulfuric smells. He first perfected his act in the French provinces but in no time was on the stage in Paris and performing around the world. He was the major attraction at the Moulin Rouge from 1892 to 1914, a beautiful theater and performance venue that was known internationally for its edgy, risqué shows.[3]

Americans ask if such a show as Le Pétomane offered on stage could be performed today. A better question: Is there anybody alive today with the unique abilities to duplicate the amazing on-stage antics of Le Péto-mane? With his anal instrumentation, Le Pétomane was able to outdraw the divine actress Sarah Bernhardt. Belgium's King Leopold II was captivated by the indescribable talents of Le Pétomane. He traveled undercover to Paris to observe his controversial demonstrations.

Le Pétomane also blew the lid off performance venues in Belgium, Spain, and North African countries. The reactions to his exhibitions in these different locales are interesting to learn from Nohain and Caradec's accounts. The authors of *Le Pétomane* describe how the Spanish authorities were outraged. The Africans were entertained and appreciative. The Arabs were scandalized and dismissed all the French as vulgar and tasteless based on the appearances of the flatulence entertainer from Paris.

Le Pétomane has an enduring legacy serving as the force behind a number of entertainment creations. He is referenced in *Blazing Saddles*, the 1974 satirical Western film by Mel Brooks. Brooks himself appears in the comedy as the dim-witted Governor William J. Le Pétomane.[4] In 1992, the Flying Karamazov Brothers premiered their play *Le Pétomane* at the La Jolla Playhouse's Mandell Weiss Forum in California. A spokesman for the Flying Karamazov Brothers proclaimed that there was "methane in their madness" in producing such a play, which drew on some "explosive material" from the original Joseph Pujol.[5]

Le Pétomane's legacy also includes musicals, such as *The Fartiste*, which was awarded Best Musical at the 2006 New York International Fringe Festival.[6] Seth Rozin's *A Passing Wind*, which premiered at the Philadelphia International Festival of Arts in 2011, also found inspiration from Le Pétomane.[7] Additionally, David Lee's 2007 reworked revival of the 1953 Broadway play *Can-Can*, which had originally been written by Abe Burroughs and Cole Porter, also drew on the life of Le Pétomane.[8] The updated play was staged at the famous Pasadena Playhouse and featured a fartiste actor with sound effects provided by a trombone and piccolo players.

Not surprisingly, British and American entertainers have tried to get in on the flatulence act since the years of the infamous Le Pétomane. In Britain, Paul Oldfield followed in Le Pétomane's "fart steps" in the 1980s as he began playing the character of Mr. Methane. At the age of 15, Oldfield realized his own abilities to fart at will while practicing yoga. He was able to develop an act of unceasing rapid-fire farts, which helped him book the opening act spots for rock bands. Mr. Methane's most accomplished cultural contribution in the world of flatulence came when he farted the British national anthem on Swedish television. He also recited Shakespeare with punctuation noises composed of flatulence.

All of Mr. Methane's rear-end capers earned him a flight in 1998 to

New York City where he appeared on *The Howard Stern Show*. Stern gathered Mr. Methane and other prominent gas passers for a competitive flatulence contest. Mr. Methane held his own—and then released his own—in the Stern competition. This opened the way for him to perform his various fart acts on Broadway. Oldfield was crowned the "British Blaster" by Stern.[9]

Howard Stern takes a backseat to no one when it comes to keeping up the flatulence entertainment tradition of the late, great Le Pétomane. Stern developed a character far more powerful than that of Mr. Methane, at least in terms of drawing a huge broadcast audience and keeping them enthralled by some novel antics. Stern's character was Fartman. Stern likened himself to a Superman of Flatulence, whose digestive system pumped foul odors into the air in the interest of truth, justice, and the American way of dealing with intestinal gas.

"I'm Fartman," Stern declared proudly in his early days of flirting with enshrinement into permanent flatulence celebrityhood. "My odorous back end whistles stinky wind in the face of adversity. I have the super sphincter that saved the planet. My brownish wind will hit my enemies in the face like doody pie."[10] Not everyone was humored by Stern's Fartman episodes or by his vaginal fart routines on his AM radio shows. The Federal Communications Commission was definitely not amused. Hollywood also resisted Stern's ideas for an *Adventures of Fartman* movie, though he was eventually successful with his box office hit, *Private Parts*, based on his autobiography of the same name published in 1993.

In his book, Stern explained that he was actually traumatized by the abdominal pain from flatulence build-up, and the embarrassment of passing gas, from an early age. At an outing to see the Rockettes at Radio City Music Hall, his father became upset with him for not letting out a few stinkers in the lobby to relieve his excruciating pain. On the way home that night, Stern said his father stopped at a rundown hotel bathroom and ordered him to fart. "Now I'm sitting in this filthy stall in this seedy hotel with my old man pacing outside the stall waiting to hear me pass gas," recalled Stern. "He's pacing, and my mother and sister are outside alone in the car."[11]

This humiliating incident from Stern's formative years does not sound like the auspicious beginnings for a superhero named Fartman who can be propelled through the air by his gas and who can use that same gas to knock evildoers unconscious. Nonetheless, Stern claims these humble beginnings launched his film, book writing, and broadcast career. In December 2015, Fartman or, rather, Howard Stern moved from terrestrial radio to SiriusXM satellite radio with a five-year contact estimated to be worth in excess of $100 million per year.

Stand Up for Flatulence

Laying cable below, above, and across America in the 1980s paved the way for a new wired television with 500-plus channels. The new cable television subsequently opened the way for fart comedians because the rationale for censorship of the airwaves was blown away. The novel technology provided an unprecedented choice in channels—and the voluntary reception of controversial content. When satellite radio came along in 1988, federal regulators also took a hands-off approach on content issues involving edgy or indecent content. Audiences agreed to receive such content—even when it was laced with noisy flatulence—with their voluntary act of paying for a regular subscription.

Comedians benefited immensely from this media expansion and the less restrictive broadcast regulatory climate. Comedians who took advantage of the new media have included George Carlin, the king of dirty words; Howard Stern, the ultimate Fartman; Eddie Murphy, who never tires of fart joke routines; Ali Wong with her insightful look at motherhood, grief, and farting; Patti Harrison, who sees farts as a needed act of resistance; and Eugene Mirman, who finds a not-so-hidden funny bone in the intestinal tract and in related bodily ailments.

George Carlin began his stand-up comedy career in the late 1950s as a fairly conventional and mild-mannered comic. This should come as no surprise on learning that Carlin's youthful idol was

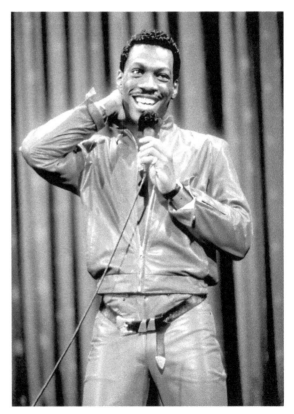

Eddie Murphy's comedy career hit a high note in 1983 with his routine about a childhood "fart game" in the family bathtub. His tale about the "big brown shark" emerging from his brother was an HBO special broadcast on the emerging medium of cable television (HBO/Photofest).

Danny Kaye and his ambition was to become like the song-and-dance man who gave us family entertainment and who hosted Disneyland events. Into the early 1960s, Carlin was mainstream. He offered "clean" performances and wore coats and ties on his nightclub gigs and on television. His performances ranged from spoofing TV game shows and emulating the "hippy-dippy" television weatherman as well as lampooning current movies and newscasts.[12]

All that changed when Carlin fell under the spell of the offbeat, edgy comedian Lenny Bruce. Carlin jettisoned the sports coats and ties; adopted the jeans and T-shirts of the counterculture; grew a beard and a ponytail; and began using scatological and offensive language that pushed the envelope. He was no longer tame or predictable. His freewheeling irreverence and anti-establishment rants got him into some legal difficulties, just as happened to his hero Lenny Bruce. What's more, Carlin found extreme flatulence.

Crude fart jokes became a staple of a Carlin performance. He asked audiences how a real comedy show could even happen without some prime fart jokes. Carlin began to describe beastly gas that could precipitate a public health emergency. He described farts in detail that could strip varnish off of furniture or that could end a happy marriage. He outlined strategies for releasing rectal gas intermittently in public place so as not to outrage bystanders.

As Carlin became more outrageous, he also engaged in harsh social commentary and became deadly serious at times. Critics said he had gone to the dark side. He seemed to relish long-winded descriptions of human beings falling victim to genocidal dictators, horrible natural disasters, deadly epidemics, and pandemics. A few fart jokes offered a bit of relief when sandwiched in between misanthropic or apocalyptic material.

Carlin's comedy transformation was tailor-made for the advent of new technologies with fewer content restrictions. He became a pioneer of comedy specials on cable television. These comedy specials became a regular model for other edgy stand-up comedians. The first of Carlin's 14 stand-up performances for HBO was filmed in 1977. Perhaps it was only logical that an in-depth retrospective on Carlin, who died in 2008, would find a home on HBO. A number of famous comedians expressed appreciation for Carlin's work in Judd Apatow's documentary that aired in 2022.

In the Apatow documentary, titled *George Carlin's American Dream*, comedian Jon Stewart talked about his admiration for Carlin's comedy work when he was a youngster. Stewart conceded that as a kid he was mystified by Carlin's description of a "side cheek, lift-up fart."

As Stewart became more enamored with the technique of a Carlin performance, he described his own amazement "that he would treat farting with the same level of scrutiny and language and deconstruction as he would the Pope, the Catholic Church hierarchy, the war machine."[13]

Apatow received kudos for making room in his documentary to talk about Carlin's propensity for fart humor. However, Apatow expressed some regret in a later interview that he did not address Carlin's flatulence leanings in more depth: "The only aspect of his career that I probably didn't spend enough time on was his silly, dirty, puerile material. He would spend an enormous amount of time on farts and boogers and pooping your pants, and oftentimes that was the first half of his set. Then he had more thoughtful political and philosophical ideas in his second set."[14]

According to Apatow, Carlin aimed to please audiences by doing many different styles of comedy within one set, and the fart humor fit right in as a genre in demand. It helped him to succeed by including both high and low comedy in his act. In contrast, a later stand-up comedian, Eddie Murphy, succeeded with a primary reliance on low comedy—and flatulence was very often center stage. Perhaps it's no coincidence that both Carlin and Murphy rank in the top of Comedy Central's listing of the 100 Greatest Stand-Ups of All Time.[15]

One of Murphy's most popular performances on flatulence appeared on the new cable medium HBO in 1983. At the start of his presentation, he accused someone in the audience of breaking a long-distance fart that could be smelled around the world. He then went on a harangue about dudes and their penchant for creating innumerable variations of what he called the "fart game." The fart game could take place in an elevator packed with dudes or in a living room where a dad introduces his son to all the fart fun during morning cartoons.

If you can play the fart game with your daddy, you can surely play it with your big brother or your best friend, according to Murphy. Murphy then recalled playing the fart game in the tub at home with his brother. He was having lots of fun with his G.I. Joe swimming on the water while his brother released depth charges. However, all hell broke loose when his brother accidentally released a "big brown shark." The mayhem that ensued brought his mother into the bathroom to call a halt to the fart game.

Murphy's comedy career has covered a lot more territory than fart games in the bathtub. He hosted *Saturday Night Live* and was a regular *SNL* comedy sketch member. He won acting awards and will forever be known for his versatility in a premium fart movie, *The Nutty Professor*. He has served as a voice actor, perhaps most famously as the donkey character in the DreamWorks animation movie *Shrek*. In 2015 Murphy received the Mark Twain Prize for American Humor by the John F. Kennedy Center for the Performing Arts.[16]

Both Carlin and Murphy are pioneers of flatulence comedy and their work in the area of gas-passing humor is memorable. That work also has inspired many other comedians to include flatulence as a portion of their comedy repertoire. A countless number of comedians have no problem acknowledging the influence of the flatulence pioneers on their own work.

Eugene Mirman, a comedian born in the old Soviet Union, has achieved the American Dream of every comedian with his work at comedy festivals, his stand-up work at restaurants and clubs, and his work on television. On the TV series *Bob's Burgers*, Mirman has played a kid named Gene Belcher who is transfixed by farts and is devoted to fart humor.[17]

Other male fart comedians include Sam Tallent, Adam Ray, Demetri Martin, Tim Allen, Erik Rivera, Nick Swardson, and many more. Tallent has squeezed laughs out of an "ungodly airplane fart." Martin also has capitalized on farts in the friendly skies and along the way to boarding planes. Ray has gotten comedy mileage out of his "long-distance farts" routine. Allen has made much of the importance of men igniting farts to their definition of manhood. Allen claims that lighting up farts is strictly the province of men. Women don't understand such behavior and would never ignite their own farts.

Whoopi and the Fartwomen

Women may be too intelligent to take on the unnecessary risk of flaming their own rectal gas in the service of amusing others. Nevertheless, flatulence comedy is not strictly a male pursuit, especially in recent decades. Whoopi Goldberg may be the first major female explorer in the realm of fart humor, perhaps not by choice but by a kind of divine design. Whoopi has had gas issues much of her life, which explains the origin of her stage name.[18]

Like George Carlin and a surprising number of comics, Caryn Elaine Johnson attended Catholic school before dropping out of formal learning institutions altogether. She became a comedic performer—a female entertainer named for a whoopee cushion. Her mother, Emma Johnson, did not name her daughter for the flatulating gag gift after she was born in 1955. Her stage name came in 2011. Her last name, "Goldberg," was also a later adoption, a name that Goldberg said reflects her heritage, like being Black.

According to Goldberg, the "Whoopi" stage forename was, indeed, derived from the farting gag gift. Goldberg recalled that when doing stand-up and stage work, there was usually little time for going to the bathroom or closing the restroom door when the opportunity presented itself. "So if you get a little gassy, you've got to let it go," Goldberg declared. "So people used to say to me, 'You're like a whoopee cushion.' And that's where the name came from."[19]

The bizarre name has stuck through the years. Whoopi Goldberg's comedy and movie career spans four decades and includes some of the most notable films ever made. The movies include *The Color Purple, The Long Walk Home, Ghost,* and *Sister Act.* Goldberg also will be long remembered for her voice work in such movies as *The Lion King.* She became the first Black woman to host the Academy Awards ceremony starting in 1994 with the 66th Oscars telecast. She returned to do it again in 1996, 1999, and 2002.[20]

Goldberg's Hollywood track record proves that a history of edgy flatulence

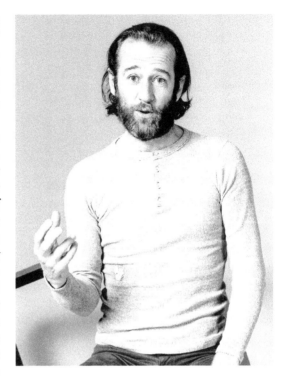

George Carlin inspired male and female comedians to turn to fart jokes for on-stage material. In his own acts, Carlin described a kind of flatulence that could strip varnish off furniture, cause temporary blindness, and doom an otherwise happy marriage (Photofest).

comedy is not a hindrance or bar to success. Goldberg has occasionally been tripped up by her controversial remarks, but she has never been down and out for the count. One of the most outrageous outbursts came at Radio City Music Hall in 2004 for a Democratic fundraiser. She pointed toward her pubic area and declared: "We should keep *Bush* where he belongs."[21] She lost work in an advertising campaign but came back to guest star in many more movies.

She also became the new moderator and co-host of television's *The View* in 2007 and is credited with boosting its viewership to 3.5 million viewers or more. Goldberg made headlines in 2014 when she interrupted a discussion about flu shots on the women's talk show. She did this with an audible cutting of the cheese. Her prominent lady discussants appeared speechless and in shock until Rosie O'Donnell began fanning the air to rid the set of any obnoxious fumes. O'Donnell's quick work to disperse Whoopi's blast elicited laughs. The entire fart event lasted less than a minute but not so in chat rooms on the Internet where it went on for days.

Goldberg apparently grossed out many men who commented on social media. Their figurative eye-rolling and complaining about her less-than-lady-like behavior were viewed by many female observers as pure sexism on the part of males. Whoopi Goldberg's long track record for flatulence comedy, and for speaking her mind on rectal gas and other subjects, may have emboldened other female comedians who picked up where she left off.

Among the increasing number of female comedians who have picked up the gauntlet to make flatulence jokes and gas humor safe for women are such performers as Ali Wong, Patti Harrison, Nikki Glaser, Hayley Georgia Morris, Jade Catta-Preta, and Michelle Wolf. Some of the younger female comics do not hold back when doing stand-up. They opine about the potency of yoga farts, about their enjoyment of letting their farts marinate under bed covers, and about outrageous "lady farts" that require a female perpetrator to leave a party in haste or to jump from a cruise ship.

The future of fart comedy may well be in the hands, and rectums, of young female comedians who howl about society's double standard when it comes to gender and flatulence. Jade Catta-Preta is one of the new female comics who concentrates on pop culture and girl power.[22]

She expresses existential angst when she explains how in the middle of the night she must leave her boyfriend's bed and quietly pass gas in the bathroom. However, when she returns to bed, her impolite boyfriend is waiting to release farts on her, whether he is awake or sleeping.

Count Nikki Glaser among the female comedians who have grown tired of the traditional expectations for women when it comes to flatulence. Women are not to be seen—and definitely not to be heard—when it comes to their gas passing or even just their feelings about farting. "It's nice to hear that people relate to the things I am talking about," said Glaser. "Women are expected to be dainty and not make fart jokes, but people come to me after shows and say, 'you sound just like me and my friends,' and that makes me feel good because sometimes I think my thoughts are a little weird."[23]

Alexandra Dawn "Ali" Wong is an Asian American comic who has gained popularity for her Netflix stand-up specials *Baby Cobra*, *Hard Knock Wife*, and *Don Wong*. She said she does not accept the notion that Asians are too reserved and cannot be funny. When it comes to her own outrageous comic sensibility, she puts the blame—or the credit—on her father: "Asians are known for being obsessed with saving face, but when my dad had to pass gas, he didn't care," she said. "In the quietest, most inappropriate places, in a church or a library or during someone's speech, he would rip it up. It was kind of great comedic timing."[24]

Patti Harrison has made giant strides in the humor business as the first big "trans comedian," though she doesn't want to be pigeonholed as a transgender or overtly political comedian. When President Donald Trump vowed to ban transgender people from the military in 2017, *The Tonight Show Starring Jimmy Fallon* invited Harrison, then 26, to share her thoughts. Harrison chided the president, saying, "Donald, you are so stupid, you are *sooo* stupid. You're lucky you're so hot." The appearance was a hit. However, Harrison said she values fart jokes as much as she does the importance of trans rights. "I love to create very dumb and stupid shit," Harrison told *Rolling Stone*. "And that's the funny thing—when people seek me out as this like political comedian, I literally just want to joke about IBS (irritable bowel syndrome) and farting."[25]

Women may be the future of flatulence comedy because they have a fresh perspective and an appreciation for the power of farting, whereas male jokesters on such vulgar matters have grown stale, trite, and predictable. Gender inequities involving the right to fart may well be the immediate future of flatulence comedy—and that is a niche for the new female comedians. In the long term, there are other promising avenues to be explored. Some of these new uncharted comedic paths lead to discussions on weird fetishes regarding flatulence.

For example, a fetish that has recently come out of the closet involves eproctopophilia, which is the term used for someone who is aroused by flatulence. Eproctophiles, especially males, reportedly spend inordinate amounts of time thinking about farting and having sexual fantasies about flatulence. Some men dream of being dominated by a really gross fart, rather than just coping with a meek poot. For female comedians who have sarcastically joked for years about the demands made upon them to be sexually submissive for men, the new demands presented by eproctophilia provide unfathomable possibilities for a comic response.

CHAPTER 9

Farts in Film

Memorable Masterpieces

Movies have capitalized on cheap laughs from moving bowels and breaking wind for decades. Sure, farting is juvenile and immature when someone rips one off on the big screen, but it's boffo box office. Critics never grow tired of slamming these films for poor taste, but audiences never grow tired of slamming the inside of a Cinema 8 to see the latest fart movies. Among the movies with memorable flatulence scenes are *The Nutty Professor, Caddyshack, Austin Powers: International Man of Mystery, Naked Gun, Harold and Kumar Go to White Castle,* and *South Park: Bigger, Longer and Uncut.* Of course, the all-time classic, which is a rite of passage and required viewing for many American males, is *Blazing Saddles* with its famous "campfire scene."

There are so many fart movies out there that some critics have taken to listing their top ten flatulence films. This study takes a more sophisticated approach by simply listing the many fart movies in specific categories. The classifications are comparatively easy to make and they beg such questions as: What movie actually has produced the best fart bubble scene with appropriate special effects? Should blue flame movies even be a category since these films may encourage adolescents to engage in risky behavior?

With the numerous fart film categories presented here, scholars and dedicated fans of flatulence movies can easily assemble several weeks of fart movie-watching. In the process, they can make their own judgments about the quality of the select offerings. At the end of each week, viewers can decide which movie won that week's category. After several months of analysis, viewers can then stack up the winners from each week and award the best overall winner in the genre of flatulence movies. This is not such an easy task and does require some rigorous analysis as well as thoughtful discussion.

At the risk of prejudicing the decision-making in the rating of the best flatulence movies of all time, this writer confesses a soft spot for the 1997 comedy film *Rain Man* and the 2019 blockbuster *The Lion King* a close runner-up. There will be plenty of naysayers with the selection of the adult offering *Rain Man* because of so many other worthy and boisterous contenders. The selection of the inspiring *The Lion King* as runner-up, easily the best children's flatulence movie, is likely to be a less contentious choice. In any case, there will be more impressive fart movies just around the corner that will render the decision-making here totally dated.

Rain Man stands out as the best fart film—with its comic phone booth scene—precisely because it is understated and subtle. Instead of an in-your-face kind of movie full of toxic men flatulating like machine guns, the farting in *Rain Man* is silent. The autistic "Rain Man" character played by Dustin Hoffman is neither offensive nor outrageous with his gas slippage. In his innocence, he simply confesses: "Uh oh, fart … uh oh, fart." Likewise, the reaction of the exasperated Tom Cruise character, as the Rain Man's brother, is relatively nuanced and sympathetic. If only all unintentional fart indiscretions could be handled in such a civilized manner.

The Lion King stands out as the best children's movie fart offering and as an overall runner-up flatulence movie. This is because of the amazing friendship between Simba, the young lion, and his animal companion, Pumbaa, the lovely little warthog. Nothing can come between their friendship, not even a jungle barking spider or a cheek squeaker in the wild. Truth is, the warthog's gas cannot be dismissed as simply an annoying floater or drifter. His farts are legendary throughout the Pride Lands of Africa.

The Lion King song about Pumbaa sums up the little animal's problematic gas-passing well: When he was young, he could "clear the savannah after every meal." The Pumbaa song is appropriately titled "Hakuna Matata," which when translated means roughly "no worries."[1] Many of us have had a brother or a very good friend with embarrassing flatulence that could clear out a playground, a classroom, a corporate boardroom, a dining room, or an entertainment center. Instead of engaging in feigned outrage, hysteria or histrionics, might we simply respond "Hakuna Matata!" No worries!

Flatulence Films: Fart-A-Thons

Blazing Saddles: Many fart aficionados rate the campfire flatulence fart-a-thon scene in the Mel Brooks' classic as the funniest and most noteworthy gas emission scene of all time. The 1974 satire featuring Gene Wilder and Richard Pryor blew the lid off any taboos discouraging fart-a-thons in film. An over-the-top comedy, the movie doesn't just take aim at previous flatulence prohibitions, but it also targets racism with the unlikely story of a Black sheriff as a hero in an all-white town in the Old West. *Blazing Saddles* was determined to be "culturally, historically, or aesthetically significant by the Library of Congress and it became a selection for preservation in the National Film Registry."[2]

The campfire flatulence extravaganza naturally occurs when a bevy of cowboys sit around the fire eating copious amounts of that valuable staple of all chuckwagons in the Old West—beans. The bean scene kicks off with a belch, followed by a fart, and then a chorus of noisy rip-snorters. A number of the cowhands insist on standing up to propel their steaming duffies up to the stars, which does not sit well with the cook. "How 'bout some more beans, Mr. Taggert?" comes a request from a happy cowboy. "I say, you've had enough," comes the response of Mr. Taggert, who vigorously fans the fermenting air at the campsite.

Nutty Professor II: The Klumps: This bizarre production, featuring comedian Eddie Murphy playing many different roles, was panned by critics as obnoxious, unfunny, loathsome, and predictably scatological. Critics aside, the actual audiences for the 2000 film gushed with superlatives and the movie literally grossed more than $160 million worldwide. Audiences gave the film high fives for Murphy's portrayal of Sherman Klump as the Nutty Professor and his clever, if vulgar, portrayals of other essential characters. Some reviewers said the Murphy film represented a career rebound and financial success.[3]

The high point—or low point—of the film occurs at the dinner scene with the Klump family. Sherman's parents get into an animated discussion about colon cleaning, when Sherman's mother suggests that the procedure is worth considering. Papa Klump expresses his skepticism and contempt for the colon cleaning idea by illustrating how he can be a do-it-yourselfer right at the dinner table when it comes to a little colon cleansing. He also suggests that Mama Klump might want to take her own hind end up to the car wash. He then carries on a marathon fart session that only concludes when Papa Klump realizes he needs to change his pants before continuing his dinner.

The Hollywood Knights: This is the ultimate frat boy movie reflecting a 1960s and 1970s mindset for practical jokes, crass behavior, and outrageous pranks. Robert Wuhl is the charismatic Hollywood Knights fraternity leader who finds support in stars Tony Danza and Michelle Pfeiffer. The Knights haze their fraternity pledges with such antics as leaving them naked in the dangerous Watts district of Los Angeles. They are chased by police officers Clark and Bimbeau who occasionally catch them to lecture them about their juvenile behavior.

Robert Wuhl's character New Bomb Turk in the Knights engages in a fantastical musical fart-a-thon when he appears at the high school pep rally. He gets up on stage to sing a rowdy rendition of the Italian favorite "Volare." However, Turk improvises with his butt. At every break in the lyrics, he pauses to break wind into the pep rally microphone. Soon, the students are having the time of their lives as their gymnasium has been turned into the original animal house. And soon, Turk is being chased around the gym by the cops and outraged school officials.

Step Brothers: Eddie Murphy was unable to restrain himself when it came to inserting an unforgettable fart occurrence in the sequel to the *Nutty Professor*. Likewise, comedian Will Ferrell was unable to resist including an endearing and enduring fart episode in the film about two grown men forced to live together as brothers. Ironically, the lengthy flatulence event originates not with Ferrell but with his brother played by John C. Reilly.

Director Adam McKay, along with Ferrell and Reilly, decided to go big with their film flatulence. They produced one of the longest farts in film history with Reilly doing the honors. Reilly's barn burner is clocked at 15 seconds. Ferrell and Reilly are job applicants in tuxedos being interviewed by an admiring character played by Seth Rogen. Rogen's admiration turns to utter disgust as Reilly unleashes his long and lingering prostate poof. "Onion and ketchup," declares Rogen as he claims to taste the unwanted fart. Hamburger accompaniments are not as explosive as baked beans, lentils, or brussels sprouts, but the aromatic condiment combination can certainly K.O. the brothers' job possibilities.

Brain Donors: Three absolute lunatics team up in this 1992 farcical comedy to run a ballet company in order to fulfill the wish of the deceased tycoon Oscar Winterhaven Oglethorpe. The ballet company is founded in his name by his widow, Lillian Oglethorpe. The lunatics who try to run the ballet operation are composed of an ambulance-chasing lawyer, a handyman, and a cab driver. Some critics trashed the film as complete and total nonsense, but other commentators praised *Brain Donors* as slapstick from another era of authentic comedy.

The fart-a-thon scene in *Brain Donors* involves an incomparable ballet dance that could have been the brainstorm of the creators of the Three Stooges or maybe the Marx Brothers. The fart scene may not involve real flatus but instead the outrageous sounds of a strategically placed whoopee cushion. The whoopee cushion can be found in the tights of the ballet performer, Volare, and the noxious noises seem to be the perfect accompaniment to the blockbuster ballet performance, if you are all in for that kind of thing.

Idiocracy: A real stinker at the box office, the 2006 science fiction comedy which zeroes in on the "dumbing down" of the world has become a popular cult film. The movie appears to draw on some ideas from H.G. Wells' *Time Machine* and Aldous Huxley's *Brave New World*. However, its premise is based on five centuries of intelligent people choosing not to have children, while the least intelligent procreate like rabbits. This results in ever dumber generations of people. The movie may actually have more in common with *The March of the Morons* by Cyril M. Kornbluth than with the classic works of Huxley or Wells.

Partisans of *Idiocracy* appreciate its takedown of brainless television programming and the relentless commercialism that exploits the dim-witted masses. The most celebrated scene in the film has to be the one in which the museum of art has been transformed into a museum of flatulence. Maya Rudolph, who plays Rita the sex worker, is on a hopeless quest to visit an art museum. No one she consults with seems to know what she is talking about. Art? She must mean fart. Finally, a well-meaning oaf explains that she is looking for the fart museum. At the museum, Rudolph pushes the explanation buttons for the exhibited artwork and is met with the sounds of farting sculptures and paintings. It's all a bit surreal. Clearly, this is not your mom and dad's museum of art.

Potent Poo Disasters

Bridesmaids: Some comedies and horror movies can't seem to decide whether they want to be about massive expulsions of flatulence or never-ending explosions of diarrhea. Why not split the difference and have plenty of both? That certainly is the unappetizing solution in *Bridesmaids*, which has a whole lot of something for everybody as the future bridesmaids go out shopping for gowns for a wedding. A major mistake for the bridal party is their dining at a spicy Brazilian restaurant before going to try on gowns at a swanky bridal shop. Farting, diarrhea, and food poisoning ensue.

Boffo buttocks performances are put in by all the talented women in this film, but no one is the equal of Melissa McCarthy. It's all over when she starts gagging, gasping, and farting in a bridal fitting room. She rushes into the elegant shop's restroom, where the porcelain throne is monopolized by a barfing bridesmaid. McCarthy has no choice but to slide down her rompers and totally desecrate a once-spotless wash basin. McCarthy fills the tiny restroom with fire-in-the-hole farts and the unwholesome sounds of a Niagara Falls of diarrhea filling the sink rim to the brim. Meanwhile, the bride-to-be is out in the middle of the street where she appears to be laying an egg—doing her business in the midst of honking horns and angry drivers.

Needless to say, this 2011 raunchy comedy was a resounding success. It became Judd Apatow's top-grossing film production. *Bridesmaids* was nominated for both an Academy Award for Best Supporting Actress for McCarthy and Best Original Screenplay for Kristen Wiig and Annie Mumalo. According to reviewer Roger Ebert, the film "definitely proves that women are the equal of men in vulgarity, sexual frankness, lust, vulnerability, overdrinking, and insecurity.... Love him or not, Judd Apatow is consistently involved with movies that connect with audiences."[4]

Harold & Kumar Go to White Castle: Harold and Kumar always connect with a specific audience: the stoner crowd. The plot for this 2004 movie is so convoluted, it is impossible to explain unless you are seriously high. The only thread that holds this disaster together is that the boys want to find themselves at a White Castle to consume some belly bombers—a sure formula for some excessive gas.

The saving grace or redemption for *Harold & Kumar Go to White Castle* comes with the inglorious poo scene. Harold and Kumar take refuge in a girls' restroom during a chase by security guards. By coincidence, they spy two hot girls whom they would like to get to know. However, they sour on the girls when they end up having to go to the bathroom—badly and bigly—as a result of a round of tacos. The girls take advantage of their unwanted fire power by playing an old camp game called "battle shits."

This poo game is among the grossest episodes in the history of fart movies, particularly from the auditory standpoint. The two girls strain on their respective toilet seats and make farting noises that would put a Brontosaurus to shame. Even Harold and Kumar grow faint as they hide in an adjacent stall and listen to the disgusting display of forced flatulence and excretions. The crowning moment comes when one of the lovely flatulating contestants concedes an end to hostilities with her declaration "Damn, you sunk my battle shit!"

Scary Movie 4: Fans of the *Scary Movie* horror film series will swear that there's a fart scene in each one of them. Who would bet against that contention? A bet worth taking is that the fart scene in *Scary Movie 4* released in 2006 is the one most notable for its total weirdness and being cleverly stupid.[5] For that matter, the fourth installment in the whole franchise series may be the weirdest. It includes a U.S. president addicted to reading *My Pet Duck*; a super weapon used by aliens to render everyone at a United Nations meeting stark naked; and an attack on Oprah on the set of the *Oprah Winfrey Show*.

The weird fart scene involves a blind girl who thinks she is in the privacy of her home but who actually is at a village meeting. She strips off most of her clothing and proceeds to relieve herself in a noisy, squeaky, gaseous manner. This is quite scary—and given the size of the audiences for this movie and its multi-million dollar box office, it's even scarier.

American Pie: In yet another poo disaster fart movie, *American Pie* again delivers the goods. The 1999 coming-of-age sex movie is all about the need to lose one's virginity before high school graduation, which supposedly is an adolescent ritual as American as apple pie. Despite the movie's financial success, most credible reviewers found it shallow, sick, awful, and without redeeming social value. Jim Sullivan of the *Boston Globe* declared *American Pie* to be a "gross and tasteless high school romp with sentimental mush."[6]

Among the many gross and tasteless scenes in *American Pie* is the "shit-break incident" when the character named Finch has to go to the potty very badly and finds his way to the girls' bathroom. He ends up making gas noises and producing a brown geyser out of his hind end. It's bad enough when this happens in the privacy of a stall in the correct bathroom, but when it happens where your girl classmates are gathered and can hear and witness it, well, that's downright mortifying. However, there are so many mortifying incidents in *American Pie*, so what's the difference?

Great Balls of Flatus Fire

Dumb and Dumber: The blue flame genre of Hollywood fart scenes is limited but potent and powerful. Blue flamers involve lighting up a gassy fart with a match for a quick flash of anal lightning. This practice is not recommended by health professionals. When Jim Carrey launched a blue flame as Lloyd Christmas in the 1994 comedy *Dumb and Dumber*, he may also have launched his movie career as one of the funniest film characters of the 1990s. Carrey as Christmas and Jeff Daniels as Harry Dunne combine as two dumb but well-meaning friends to make box office gold. The movie proved to be a hot commodity and spawned a commercially successful prequel in 2003 and a popular sequel in 2011.

Carrey's repertoire of farting in *Dumb and Dumber* is extensive and includes an explosive incident after his drink is spiked with a laxative by his close friend. The character played by Jeff Daniels is apparently trying to sabotage Carrey's date with a girl named Mary. Later, Carrey is daydreaming of being with Mary at a winter party. He decides to entertain the crowd at the winter party by lifting his legs far over his head. Carrey's feat of gymnastics amazes the party, which is then totally wowed when he brandishes a lighter near his posterior and ignites a fart. Despite the wild approval of the revelers in *Dumb and Dumber*, this kind of entertainment should not be tried at home with mom and dad—or even a frat house winter party.

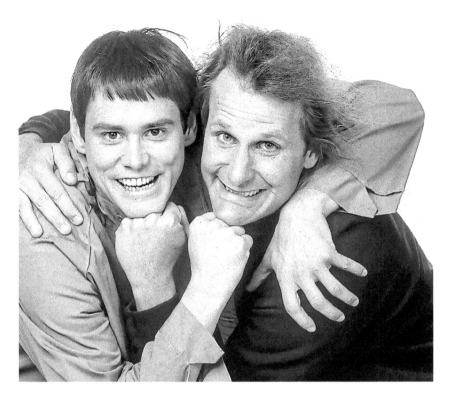

Jim Carrey (left) and Jeff Daniels play Lloyd Christmas and Harry Dunne, two intellectually-challenged friends, in the comedy film *Dumb and Dumber* (2014). Naturally, the film boasts a memorable and fiery "blue dart" fart scene by Carrey (New Line Cinema/Photofest).

South Park: Bigger, Longer and Uncut: Those nasty *South Park* kids have given us an adult comedy feature movie released by Comedy Central, much to the dismay of mothers and fathers. Many moms and dads feel the characters corrupt their children and coarsen the culture. In fact, this 1999 film parodies "bad parenting" and satirizes moralistic attempts at censorship. The plot is unusually twisted even by *South Park* standards. The blue flame fart scene is inspired when the characters Stan, Kyle, Cartman, and Kenny witness a blue flame fart scene at a movie called *Asses of Fire*.

The children are reprimanded for seeing the forbidden movie. *Asses of Fire* is blamed for the children's cussing profusely at school, so they are sent to the school counselor and to a special class to address their obsession with the movie and its profanity. The class and counseling session fail miserably because shortly afterward Cartman bets Kenny that he cannot set a fart on fire. Kenny imitates the movie scene and sets himself on fire with his fart. He is rushed to the hospital, where a doctor accidentally replaces his heart with a baked potato, which subsequently explodes and kills him. Cartman's parents ground him, while Kenny ends up in hell with Satan for his misbehavior. Satan torments Kenny and his new partner in the hell fires, a recent arrival named Saddam Hussein.

Joy of Sex: This ill-fated 1984 film was allegedly based on the best-selling sex manual by Alex Comfort. The Hollywood masterminds felt the movie could be about anything and be successful because it was associated with the title of the popular sex education book. Critics argued that the movie was about nothing and rightly destined to be a box office failure. Reviewers trashed it for its reliance on sex and other bodily functions. Even the movie's director, Martha Coolidge, said she had to answer yes to these questions: Will the film "embarrass me, humiliate me, disgust me for the rest of my life?"[7]

Ironically, it's those "other bodily functions" movie excerpts that ensure the *Joy of Sex* will be remembered and cherished, especially by teen boys. A specific tantalizing scene involves male teens packed in a car and acting up in front of a drive-in movie screen. The boys brag about who has eaten the most fart-producing foods, including Brussels sprouts, beans, artichokes, and Swedish meatballs. A boy in the car with a Slavic accent innocently asks: "What is this blue flames?" The fellows quickly produce their cigarette lighters and the flaming begins. When the driver sets himself on fire, the drive-in moviegoers on either side of the offensive boys fire up their engines, announce their total disgust, and quickly drive away. However, the actual audiences for this move stayed for more.

Fragrant Methane Bubbles

Last Action Hero: Arnold Schwarzenegger plays a ruthless assassin, Jack Slater, in this 1993 action comedy and also was the film's co-producer. The film is full of police chases, heinous crimes, and vile mobsters, but what truly sets it apart is a fart bubble. A fart bubble occurs when gas is emitted below the surface of a liquid, usually water in a tank or a hot tub, and then finds its way to the surface where it pops with a powerful pungency. In addition to the unique fart bubble, the Schwarzenegger movie is noted as comedian Art Carney's last feature film before his death in 2003.[8]

The fart bubble scene occurs when Slater shows up at the funeral of mobster "Leo the Fart" at the top of a hotel slammed with mafia folks.

A particularly clever mobster plants a nerve gas bomb in the cadaver so when it releases gas, the explosion will kill everyone in its vicinity. Slater is on to the conspiracy and hustles the body out of the funeral under the pretense that Leo is still breathing—and still farting. The deceased ends up in a tar pit where the definitively dead Leo passes gas one last time and it surfaces safely as a giant fart bubble from the pit. Apologies for this spoiler to anyone inspired to see the movie of Jack Slater and Leo the Fart.

Hot Shots! Part Deux: This 1993 poof spoof is packed with star power, including Lloyd Bridges, Charlie Sheen, Valeria Golino, Richard Crenna, Brenda Bakke, Miguel Ferrer, Rowan Atkinson, and Jerry Haleva. Sheen takes on the role of a would-be Rambo and Bridges is the president of the United States. The plot involves an American special forces team that gets in trouble when invading Saddam Hussein's palace in Iraq. The mission to rescue captured U.S. soldiers from Operation Desert Storm unravels and a retired CIA agent with special skills is called out of retirement to save the day.

Lloyd Bridges as President Benson becomes part of the secret mission to Iraq and his fart scene stands out as one of the seminal sea scenes in this financially successful farce of a movie. While the president is scuba diving in the ocean, an Iraqi patrol boat runs over the swimmers in the water. A previous presidential lunch hits his stomach as he traverses underwater and a series of executive farts result. The silent-but-deadly fart bubbles head to the surface and release a killer gas upon the Iraqis—and the mission continues. Bridges was nearing age 80 at the time of the fart and movie, which lends some credence to the capabilities for fermented gas production.[9]

Austin Powers International Man of Mystery: This is the first installment in the dramatic comedy spy series of movies featuring Mike Myers. He plays a James Bond character who thwarts the terrible conspiratorial activities of Dr. Evil. This time the evil doctor hatches a plot to steal nuclear weapons and blackmail the world for a ransom of $1 million. He jacks up his demand to a sum of $100 billion when he discovers the impact of inflation on the U.S. dollar.

Just like James Bond, Austin Powers is enjoying the ladies when he is not tripping up the bad guys. In the case of this spy thriller, Austin Powers enjoys the company of the sexpot Alotta Fagina in a hot tub. He becomes so excited that he slips with an unintended fart release. Instead of being disgusted by what normally would be considered crude behavior, Fagina gets turned on when Austin Powers' fart bubbles find freedom in the hot tub. However, this kind of reaction is probably only possible when peculiar sex goddesses like Fagina are in the presence of a James Bond or an Austin Powers. So don't get any ideas, fellas.

Blame a Duck for It

Caddyshack: Only teen boys and young males are likely to want to take credit for an egg sandwich fart or a heavy, brown ale fart. Most people are likely to blame an errant fart on the snoozing bloodhound in front of the fireplace—while the hound is digesting his favorite meal of horse meat and fatty gravy. There are other options besides blaming the dog. *Caddyshack* is the landmark comedy that instructs us to blame that noisy rat-a-tat, quack-quack gaseous emission on a hapless duck passing through the neighborhood.

The film's reception in 1980 was less than stellar, as critics used the usual harsh adjectives. Despite a classic fart incident, critics described the movie as crude, vulgar, juvenile, and disgusting.[10] First-time film director Harold Ramis also came in for criticism for a disorganized plot and only average comic routines. However, Rodney Dangerfield's and Bill Murray's appearances were singled out for praise. As the film has ripened with age, and with a collection of reappraisals over the years, both Dangerfield and Murray have been cited in this golf cult classic as rendering above-par performances.

The memorable fart scene occurs when the Dangerfield character is wearing an obnoxious plaid sport coat and begins bragging about his real estate prowess. He appears to be in a swanky golf club dining area with rich clientele. They are only mildly interested in his bombastic declaration of faith in real estate over the stock market. He startles everybody when he leans to one side at the table and rips off the mightiest meat fart ever to wrinkle the drapes of a country club. He follows the fart with the famous line that will live in infamy: "Oh, did somebody step on a duck!" The line has immortalized Dangerfield.

Spies Like Us: Chevy Chase and Dan Aykroyd play two expendable spies acting against the old Soviet Union. They are meant to act as decoys to draw attention away from more competent secret agents. This Cold War comedy shows how two novice intelligence agents, who lack in the intelligence department, are still capable of preserving the American way of life. In fact, after their success in staving off a nuclear war, the two stars become nuclear disarmament negotiators.

Chevy Chase becomes embroiled in a fart scene that employs his best comedic skills to maximum effect. Those skills also allow him to effectively cast blame for his obnoxious gas passing. Chase tries to cheat on a government exam employing every scam in the book. He attempts to bribe the instructor; he wears an eye patch with the answers written on its inside; he distracts attention when the exam begins. He lets go with a loud fart that has the entire class looking to the back of the room. Chase successfully makes faces and gestures that shift the blame for the fart to the "sitting duck" in the desk across from him.

Phone Booth and Elevator Farts

Rain Man: Everyone of reasonable age and average olfactory skills will know the distress of being stuck in a small space in stagnant air tainted by a rumper trumper, a fanny frog, or butt sneeze. A dressing room can be polluted with a lingering trouser cough. A fast-food restroom can be nauseating with the remains of an ass droid or a crank bug. An elevator space can be defiled by a hot cheese bubbler or brown growler. In the 1997 classic *Rain Man*, actor Tom Cruise suffers the indignity of being stuck in a phone booth with a silent wet one proffered by Dustin Hoffman, who plays an autistic savant.

Cruise is the shyster, wheeler-dealer Charlie Babbitt. Hoffman plays the role of Raymond, whose autism has resulted in his confinement to a mental institution most of his life. Charlie discovers that his deceased father has willed the family estate to Raymond. Charlie was unaware that he even had a brother, but he quickly tries to become his best friend on a cross-country road trip. Charlie hopes to gain custody of Raymond, the Rain Man, to gain control of the money. A lot goes wrong on the brothers' road trip together, but a few things go right as Charlie develops a love for his long-lost brother.

One of the things that goes wrong is when Charlie makes a desperate call in a phone booth, where he keeps Raymond close to keep him from wandering away. As the Cruise character gets a whiff of the flatus that Raymond has released, he becomes genuinely exasperated with his savant brother. "Did you fart?" Charlie interrogates his brother, who innocently repeats, "Uh oh, fart." When Cruise asks his brother how he can stand it, while struggling to open the phone booth door, the Rain Man simply responds: "I don't mind."

Police Academy 5: Assignment Miami Beach: Of all the movies in the *Police Academy* series, the fifth installment may be the most despised and denigrated film by critics and audiences alike. Gene Siskel of the *Chicago Tribune* gave the film zero stars and stated, "I didn't laugh once during the entire film—not at the slapstick, not at the humor, which is pitched at the preschool level."[11] If there is one small saving grace for this movie about the Miami Police Department, it may be the elevator fart scene.

Sure, there are as many farts in the *Police Academy* series of movies as there are donuts made daily, destined for the men in blue. However, the fart left in an elevator by a kidnapper of Commandant Eric Lassard has found a permanent place in the minds of academy audiences. Flatulence enthusiasts will recall how both kidnappers and the commandant move to one side of the elevator to isolate the truly guilty party. Cops and crooks alike have little tolerance for inconsiderate flatulating in a closed space.

Liar, Liar: Jim Carrey has starred in plenty of movies that have made money but have been dismissed as trite, superficial, and forgettable. *Liar, Liar* is not one of those movies. The box office for the 1997 film approached a third of a billion dollars. Critics gave it positive reviews and Carrey was called the "laughable lawyer" character and was nominated for Best Actor in a Comedy at the 56th Golden Globe Awards.[12] Perhaps the premise was the "deal-maker" for the film: A longtime lying lawyer finds himself "cursed" for just one day to speak only the truth. This uncomfortable situation for the attorney, who must only tell the truth, shocks his family and jeopardizes his career.

Carrey, as Los Angeles attorney Fletcher Reede, must even own up to his own elevator fart as his excruciating day of truth takes a toll on him. After ripping off a silent but monstrous fart in the office elevator, he leaves four suffering beings behind who are fanning the air, pinching their nostrils, and wavering on their feet. Before the doors on the compartment can close, he turns around and declares to them in a very loud voice: "It was me!" He owns up to his indiscretion. His honesty is refreshing—but apparently the only thing that is refreshing.

Revenge Farts and Fart Bullies

Click: Passing gas is not always an indiscretion, an unintended slip-up, or a physical imperative that can no longer be bottled up or restrained. Sometimes passing sulfuric gas is malevolent and intentional. Sometimes it's an act of toxic masculinity; an act of insidious revenge; or an act of a no-holds-barred bully. In *Click*, actor Adam Sandler uses a pent-up fart to punish the boss whom he so despises and wishes to demean. By a crucial twist of fate, Sandler's character can do this with impunity.

Adam Sandler plays Michael Newman, an overworked architect who is bullied by his boss. As a dedicated professional, Newman often has to neglect his wife and kids to handle his work load. One day he visits a Bed Bath & Beyond store to buy a universal remote and accepts a magical remote provided free by a scientist and experimenter. Architect Newman engages in some crass mischief, but what also unfolds in this 2006 comedy is a cross between the *Time Machine* and the *Wizard of Oz*.

In the revenge fart scene, Newman enters his boss's office with a magical remote that can manipulate time, including freezing it and fast-forwarding it. Newman resents his boss who happens to be David Hasselhoff playing the character of John Ammer. Newman uses the remote to freeze his over-bearing boss so that he can punch him and rough him up. Then he positions his rump in his boss's face and lets a powerful fart fly. When time resumes, Ammer wakes up and wonders aloud why his mouth tastes so nasty. Newman has successfully executed a revenge fart on Ammer, courtesy of his ready rump and his magical remote.

Can't Buy Me Love: Not even a thousand dollars can buy the love of a teen girl, but the offer can get her attention. In this 1987 teen romance movie, a nerd at a high school in Tucson, Arizona, gives popular cheer-leader, Cindy, the money to be his girlfriend for a month. Nerdy Ronald trades his geeky friends for cool students. He has a clothing and hair makeover under Cindy's care. Cindy eventually decides to hang out with Ronald rather than her popular friends. Ronald asks Cindy to the prom and they kiss for the first time. As the Beatles' title song plays, the happy couple rides off into the sunset on Ronald's ride-on lawn mower.

Although the little brother of the nerdy protagonist in *Can't Buy Me Love* is in a subordinate role, he is a cute and extremely sympathetic character. He likes to follow his older brother around but is constantly fart-bullied by the older boys. When he finds his brother at a party and wants to check out the scene, he gets a face full of flatus from one of the older jocks. When he sneaks into the back seat of a car with the older boys, he gets another dose of the flatulence treatment. Older brother Ronald makes out like a bandit, but no amount of money can buy his little brother love from the fart bullies.

Jay & Silent Bob: This 2001 film is another stoner odyssey that has been described as a moderate commercial success. The movie is less than a moderate comedy success. The plot is convoluted and difficult to explain, much less to watch. Jason Mewes plays Jay and Kevin Smith plays Silent Bob. Critics note the excess of crude language in this production, which might have benefited by simply being a silent film.

Many comedies are all about questioning cultural norms and defying established authority. Sometimes a fart in the kisser delivers the defiant message. Jay and Silent Bob are apprehended by a police officer on suspicion of selling an illegal substance—pot. After pleading their innocence to the cop, the officer thinks he has the suspects nailed by pointing out they have rolling papers in their possession. However, the boys argue that the papers are just handy wipes for hind-end accidents, and then the officer gets a full moon and a fart in the face. For this offense, Jay and Bob should be held in contempt in a court of law and by any presiding movie audience.

Shaun of the Dead: Do zombies pass gas? This 2004 zombie comedy is a thoroughly British production, but it certainly caught the attention of American audiences. Maybe that's because the two main characters, Shawn played by Simon Pegg and his friend Ed played by Nick Frost, seem totally unaware that they are in the midst of a zombie apocalypse. The horror of the walking dead just doesn't seem to register or to pierce the fog of high intensity hangovers that afflict these two amiable idiots.

For flatulence aficionados, this movie offers the perfect illustration of the silent-but-deadly fart that can be used to bully, punk, or subjugate its victims. When Ed apologizes to Shawn in a serious moment in the film, the befuddled Shawn tells him it's all good and he shrugs his shoulders. Shawn doesn't understand why he deserves an apology from Ed. However, Ed repeats his apology more emphatically and then Shawn's face contorts, he falls backward, and he gets it. Shawn gets that he has been victimized by the ultimate silent-but-deadly fart.

Monty Python and the Holy Grail: Sometimes a fart bully can be a Frenchman in a medieval castle simply taunting an Englishman with his flatulence. Not just any old limey, however, merits such disrespect. In the Monty Python classic comedy, the British victim of the fart taunt happens to be King Arthur, surrounded by his faithful Knights of the Round Table. They happen to be traveling in quest of the holy object that is part of the Arthurian legend of the 13th century.

When King Arthur, situated below the castle walls with his knights, looks up and begins to question the French watchman, the response is one for the ages: "You don't frighten us, English pig-dogs! Go and boil your bottoms ... I don't want to talk to you no more, you empty-headed animal food trough wiper! I fart in your general direction! Your mother was a hamster and your father smelt of elderberries!"

Flatulence Outliers

Polyester: Some movie fart scenes cannot be easily pigeonholed in any particular category. They involve flatulence that is neither captured in an ascending bubble, encapsulated in a crowded elevator, nor ignited as a blue dart emerging from the buttocks. The thing that makes *Polyester* distinctive is its Odorama. The film itself is about the ennui of suburban housewives and their yearning to be rescued from their humdrum existence. This 1981 satire of the melodramatic genre of women's pictures manages to touch on divorce, alcoholism, foot fetishism, and the anger of the religious right.

The Odorama feature of the film allows viewers to smell what is found on the screen by using scratch-and-sniff cards supplied before the movie begins. The fart smell is sandwiched in between roses and airplane glue.

The Odorama gimmick was inspired by the 1960 work of William Castle for *Scent of Mystery*. That film featured a device dubbed as "Smell-O-Vision." The gimmick for *Polyester* was an invention for the cinema advertised with the tagline "It'll Blow Your Nose!"[13]

The Naked Gun: From the Files of Police Squad!: Detective Frank Drebin, played by Leslie Nielsen, became the master of crime comedy films in America in the last century. In *The Naked Gun* installment of 1988, Drebin is on the job sleuthing a conspiracy to assassinate Queen Elizabeth II who is on a state visit to the United States. There has been plenty of farting in Nielsen's many detective films, but often the farting is difficult to classify.

Such is the case with *The Naked Gun: From the Files of Police Squad!* It's just hard to classify. In this movie, Nielsen is in the john, but he is not creating a disaster poo fart scene; it's a pee fart scene that makes it unique. His character, Frank Drebin, is taking a long pee in the urinal after speaking at a press conference. Drebin forgets that he still has his microphone on and the entire audience for the next press conference speaker can hear his splashing, his singing, and the flatulence that he lets rip as his urination session comes to an end.

Swiss Army Man: This film is classified as an absurdist black comedy for good reason. It premiered at a Sundance Film Festival in 2016.[14] In order to understand this movie, think about the 2000 Tom Hanks movie *Cast Away*, in which Hanks is marooned on an island and makes friends with a soccer ball that washes up. In the case of *Swiss Army Man,* the marooned Hank Thompson, played by Paul Dano, is amused when a farting cadaver washes up.

The bubbly farts propel the cadaver across the water and it never seems to run out of gas. At one point, Hank climbs up on the floating corpse and rides it across the ocean like a jet ski. The two of them end up on a mainland shore, but they are still far from civilization. Some members of the audience for this film at its first Sundance showing thought it was less than civilized. They thought the premise was outrageous and walked out on the film.[15]

Mystery Men: The Spleen: Another terminally weird movie, this 1999 superhero comic film is being called a cult classic, but even that designation is charitable at best. The film has an impressive cast which includes Ben Stiller, Paul Reubens, William H. Macy, Greg Kinnear, Janeane Garofalo, Tom Waits, and more. Tom Waits is the mad scientist Dr. Heller, who devises non-lethal weapons for use by the Mystery Men.

A fatal flaw for *Mystery Men: The Spleen*, according to most critics, is that the entire movie comes off as one giant fart joke. Paul Reubens plays The Spleen, a superhero character who can vanquish all enemies with his sonic ass gas. Some people find the movie trite and monotonous. In the movie's defense, The Spleen does offer an assortment of volleys from his gaseous weaponized butt. Sometimes he renders a potent, noisy blast, while other times he switch hits, employing a silent-but-deadly shot of flatulence.

Gas Planet: Okay. Cut these short fart movie reviews some slack. This movie, an abbreviated work, merits only a short one-paragraph review, but it does deserve some mention in passing. The 1992 film is animated and has received criticism for not being up to the pixel standards of a movie like *Toy Story*, which actually came out three years later. Three bizarre-looking bird-like creatures inhabit this production. They pop around their planet eating gas balls and then have no choice but to fart. It's a nice, goofy offering for kids and adults who have not grown up, presumably a lot of people reading this book.

The Lighthouse: There are enough gaseous farts in this 2019 movie to supply blue dart flames to guide all the ships at sea. The film is about two lighthouse keepers who appear to go mad as a storm maroons them on the tiny island where they are stationed. Ephraim Winslow, played by Robert Pattinson, is a contract lighthouse keeper. Thomas Wake, played by Willem Dafoe, is the older and more experienced lighthouse keeper. Things go less than swimmingly, with poor Wake killed by an axe at movie's end, while Winslow is seen naked on the rocky beach with gulls pecking at his exposed bowels.

Excessive farting by both Wake and Winslow is among the many things that rub the two lighthouse keepers the wrong way. The younger Winslow is especially put off by the salty old dog's habit of farting at meal time. When Winslow later reciprocates with a few methane bombs of his own, the crusty old-timer becomes enraged and appears to be offended at what looks like a case of one-upmanship. They increasingly cross swords, especially when there is "dirty weather knocking about." The weather stinks. Everything stinks. There's just not enough room in this lighthouse for these two flatulating fools.

Goldmember: The Mike Myers spy comedy satirizing *Goldfinger* may be superior to the original spy movie thanks to additional characters such as Dr. Evil, Gillian Shagwell, Fook Yu, Fook Mi, Mini-Me and, of course, Fat Bastard. When Fat Bastard lets a wet one rip in the presence of Austin Powers, the super spy must ask in disgust: "Did you just soil yourself?" The chubby character then goes into an analysis and commentary about his flatulence. He waves his hands and cheers, "wafting, wafting," as he waves his arms. He observes that "everyone likes their own brand, don't they? This is magic." Austin Powers seems to lose all his super powers when Fat Bastard declares that his output smells of "carrots and throw up" and would easily "gag a maggot."

Like Water for Chocolate: This 1992 Mexican romantic drama is a nice contrast to the bombastic Austin Powers thriller. The characters Tita and Juan de la Garza provide a needed respite from Fat Bastard and Dr. Evil. The foreign-language film is based on a 1989 novel by Mexican novelist Laura Equivel in the tradition of magical realism.[16] Tita is a dynamic woman living in the early 1990s and experiences struggles involving family traditions, romantic yearnings, economic inequality, and revolution.

The beautiful Tita is a marvelous chocolate maker and a heroine in the film on many levels, including that of therapist for the flatulating. When the character Rosaura comes into the chocolate kitchen and asks Tita for help with her diet, Tita embraces the challenge. Not only has Rosaura gotten very fat, but she also has a serious issue with flatulence and with bad breath, which drives her be-

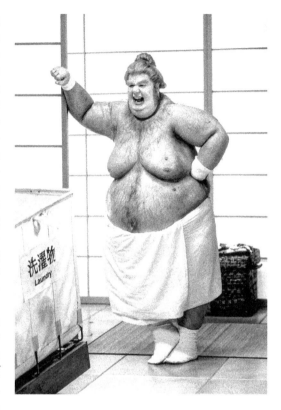

In the James Bond rip-off film *Goldmember* (2002), the heartless character known as Fat Bastard lets a wet one blast in the presence of Austin Powers. The wilting super spy, played by Mike Myers, must ask Fat Bastard, also played by Myers, in disgust: "Did you just soil yourself?" (New Line Cinema/ Photofest).

loved Pedro farther and farther away. It's clear that there's no lovemaking going on with Pedro anymore. Like a good sister, Tita promises to help her lose weight—and smell better.

Just for Kiddies?

George of the Jungle: Uncle Walt of the Disney Studios will forever be known for his extremely popular animated children's movies. Walt Disney and his films were renowned for their propriety and standards of taste.

So many adult fans raise their eyebrows and express skepticism when they learn that flatulence crept into some of the most revered family offerings. One of these was the 1997 hit *George of the Jungle*. The movie is a spoof of the Tarzan tales about a primitive young man raised in the jungle by animal friends.

The gorilla who helped raise George in the Disney film has a problem. The gorilla is a very smart primate but does not seem to have the intelligence to address an intestinal malady. (What? There are no anti-gas tabs available at the local jungle pharmacy?) The gorilla's malady provides fodder for some goofy gorilla fart jokes. Who would have guessed that Disney would be capable of fart-shaming. The poor gorilla's flatulence issues make him the butt of some silly jabs and jibes—and in front of all those children!

The Lion King: The young Lion named Simba is in line to succeed his father, the king of the Pride Lands, in this 2019 blockbuster. However, Simba's devious uncle named Skar kills Mufasa and takes the throne, while Simba runs off into exile in the jungle. Simba joins up with some carefree characters like Timon, the wise-acre meerkat, and Pumbaa, the naïve warthog that suffers from flatulence. After growing up with these outcasts, Simba gets a little wisdom from Rafiki, a mandrill shaman, that provides the impetus for Simba to challenge Skar and take his rightful place as king.

Every future king should have a farting warthog as a friend to humor him and help him find his rightful place in the hierarchy of creation. In the case of Simba, a pup of a lion, that wonderful warthog would be the exceptionally gassy Pumbaa. This magical farting warthog merits a song in the Disney blockbuster titled "Hakuna Matata" (Swahili for "no worries"). The popular song pretty well sums up the impact of Pumbaa's prodigious farting: after every meal, he could clear the savannah with it.[17]

Rocket Man: This 1997 science fiction comedy was one of those rare Disney movies that crashed big time. It failed to get off the launch pad with critics and fizzled with audiences with only a few million dollars in box office payload. The film's plot is about a shaky mission to Mars with lots of glitches. The crew makes it to Mars after eight months of hyper sleep only to encounter numerous Martian storms that put the mission in peril. A safe journey back home is marred by the realization that the American flag boxers posted on a pole on the red planet have been stolen by a Martian.

Outer space is not the ideal locale for fart explosions. NASA scientists ought to know better than to have astronauts dining on space beans while in transit. In *Rocket Man*, astronaut Harland Williams gets into trouble after dining on the favorite musical fruit of Earthlings. The beans cause a serious crisis in his spacesuit with a monstrous fart bubble threatening the viability of the air-supply tube. His NASA handlers are unconvinced when the space voyager denies that the flatulence was not his. "It wasn't me" just does not cut it on a sparsely-populated planet millions of miles from Earth.

Flubber: This 1997 science fiction comedy features Robin Williams as the crazy professor Philip Brainard of Medfield College. He wants to invent a new energy source to raise enough money to save the college from closing. His singular mission causes him to miss important appointments, including two wedding dates with his girlfriend, Sara. He finally has some success creating a sentient green goo with amazing elasticity and energy potential. Brainard calls it "Flubber." Numerous scoundrels want to steal or buy his invention. Brainard and Sara foil the bad guys; save the invention; save the college; and have a successful wedding.

The gooey mess invented by the mad professor in *Flubber* eventually transforms into a major movie character of the same name. Flubber has his own brand of high-energy flatulence that would put any mere pork-and-beans-gorging human to shame. When a movie villain tries to consume and digest Flubber, the shiny green fellow breaks wind and blasts out of his ass crack. So what's not to like with this kind of ending? Critics thought the director, writers, and actors completely flubbed it, but audiences anted up the cash for tickets and reportedly loved the green goo special effects.

Does Queefing Count?

Private Parts: Does queefing count as a fart? That's not even a serious question for Howard Stern. The New York City radio shock jock practically invented the term "pussy fart." Stern has always been happy to explain how air gets in—and air gets out of—a woman's privates to create something similar to anal-origination flatulence. In the autobiographical movie *Private Parts*, Stern recounts the start of his radio career and his many broadcasts educating listeners about the mighty winds that emanate from human orifices.

In *Private Parts*, the radio personality who aspired to be the superhero character Fartman pulls on-air stunts that get him in trouble with his broadcast bosses, the censors, and the law. In the 1997 movie, Stern has sex with a female listener by having her undress and straddle the woofer speaker in her entertainment center. Stern provides some strange radio wave audio to the woofer. His virtual sex partner enjoys the stimulation from the woofer and appears to orgasm—and it's not just the woofer that is making noise.

Heartbreak Kid: Ben Stiller stars as Eddie Cantrow in a dark romantic comedy about a hapless bachelor and sports shop owner who just can't seem to get it right when it comes to finding the kind of relationship that would make for a good marriage. When Eddie falls for Lila, played by Malin Akerman, he's convinced he's finally made the connection to happily-ever-after wedded bliss. However, when the couple honeymoon in Cabos San Lucas, he quickly realizes that he has made a colossal mistake. He can't stand her incessant singing, her newly-revealed history of drug abuse, her deviated septum, her sleep issues, and her dubious employment history.

And that's not all. Lila has a revved-up sex drive that's so wild that the Stiller character feels physical pain when making love. On top of that, she queefs just like a drunken sailor farts. After he and his new wife get finished with sex at the resort hotel, Lila excuses herself to go to the bathroom. The toilet seat comes down with a bang and then a virtual horse fart is heard. "It's not what you think it is," she declares. "I didn't hear anything," the embarrassed Eddie Cantrow responds. "I just queefed … big time," she tries to explain to him. "If you don't know what a queef is, well … google it," she adds.

CHAPTER 10

Merchandising of Fart Gifts

In the beginning, there was the whoopee cushion. The creation of this practical joke device was for the production of obnoxious, squeaky, flapping noises. These aural emission toys were meant for those who enjoy sophomoric, childish, goofy flatulence humor. Whoopee cushion enthusiasts have enjoyed fart humor for centuries. Through thick and thin, fart humorists have believed that the funny bone can be found in the anatomical vicinity of the buttocks, near where acoustic breezes exit.

Partisans of posterior repartee generally have agreed that there is no substitute for a bona fide fart, but the right invention will succeed in creating a combination of wind and noise, a bit of laughter, and a bit of humiliation for anyone pranked by this performance gadgetry. Known today by such names as the wind blaster, the poot pillow, the fart bag, and Razzberry Cushion, these items can all trace their origins to ancient times. Noblemen once relished hiding inflated animal bladders under cushions of palace furniture. Unsuspecting guests of royalty sat upon these crude whoopee cushions and embarrassed themselves in the process.

The Roman emperor Elagabalus, whom historians have identified as a royal pain in the ass, loved playing practical jokes on others. The youthful Elagabalus would place the ancient whoopee cushion implements under the cushions of palace guests he considered to be pompous. Elagabalus was emperor from 218 to 222 AD. His short reign was notorious for sex scandals, religious controversy and unhappy dinner guests. His immature behavior alienated the Roman Empire's elites and even the common people became disenchanted, so it should come as no surprise that Elagabalus was just 18 years old when he was assassinated.[1]

Many more artificial flatulence devices were used in pranks in subsequent centuries. They involved leaders who enjoyed hiding inflated animal bladders under cushions to embarrass unsuspecting guests. However, Elagabalus may be the only leader whose penchant for posterior humor led to an assassination. In the earliest years of fart humor, contraptions to simulate the expulsions of human methane were largely the province of

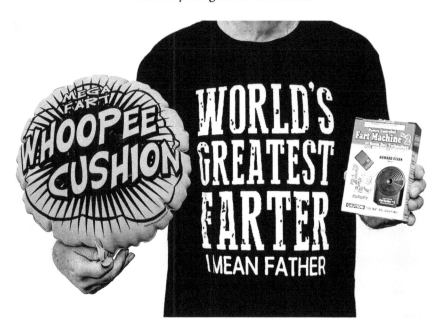

Flatulence merchandise and gag gifts can range from old-fashioned whoopee cushions to the latest remote control fart machines. Various iterations of the infamous whoopee cushion have elicited belly laughs for centuries (photograph by Ursula Ruhl).

the elites residing in the palace. This changed with the industrial revolution and the mass production of devices that could be enjoyed by the common populace. Just as shit happens, improvements happen.

A modern rubber version of the whoopee cushion was invented in the 1920s by the JEM Rubber Company of Canada using scrap sheets of rubber. A saleable version of this vulgarity was marketed with some success and became known as the "Razzberry Cushion."[2] These whoopee cushions were constructed from two sheets of rubber glued together at the edges. A small opening imitating the natural flatulating anus allowed air to enter and leave the cushion.

Initially, these contraptions could break apart easily and lacked staying power. To use these whoopee cushions, a prankster had to first inflate it with air, then place it on a chair or squeeze it manually. When it was put on a suitable piece of furniture, an unsuspecting victim would sit on the whoopee cushion, forcing air out of the constricted opening, which caused the flap to vibrate to make a loud farting sound. Despite its lack of durability and design flaws, these cushions have been enjoyed by millions and it is estimated that the imaginary farts produced by these contrivances may now number in the trillions.

Enter Microchip Farts

Modern electronics has vastly improved upon the whoopee cushion. There is no need for inflated animal bladders or rubber balloons that open and then deflate. Electronics that can produce farting noises involve oscillator circuits that at first used vacuum tubes, then transistor circuitry, and eventually miniaturized electronic chips. Semi-conductor chips powered by nine-volt batteries or penlight cells are far more reliable than the old rubber bladder devices.

Electronic hobbyists and experimenters are fond of converting synthesizer circuits into farting devices or wiring their own "bread board" circuitry. These can provide a wide range of fart noises that vastly exceed the abilities of an average sphincter. However, it is not necessary to be an electronics experimenter or microchip hobby enthusiast to enjoy the latest in fart audiology. The devices are now found as consumer products and holiday gifts, mostly online, but sometimes at consignment shops where they have been retired.

A plethora of fart gifts now mirror—or echo—the variety in acoustics often associated with flatulence. Noise makers are big sellers, from the audible farting teddy bear to the giant yellow fart button that makes 20 funny poop noises and farting sounds. For more elaborate tastes or discerning ears, there are the T.J. Wiseman Remote Control Fart Machines, the Stinky Pig Game, and the politically divisive Pull My Finger Farting Donald Trump Plush Doll with Animated Hair. Simple and crude whoopee cushions are taking a back seat to wired fart simulation devices that are described as "the bomb" by elated consumers. The number of fart gifts now available for buyers is an indication of the endless and eternal popularity of fart humor.

Remote control fart machines are leading sellers at Halloween, Christmas, Mardi Gras and St. Patrick's Day. The small devices can be operated with a controller and are best hidden in a spot near where an unsuspecting victim is likely to sit. Males are the most likely purchasers who delight in embarrassing a spouse, a brother or sister, or a father with a reputation for too often delivering the real thing. Cheap thrills also are available for those desiring to "punk" the family dog. For those unwilling to confine such humor to the family circle, co-workers or even sad sack bosses in the workplace can become easy targets.

Perfect strangers visiting coffee shops also have suffered the indignity of pranksters who place the device in a large envelope or inside a winter coat stashed on an adjacent chair. The perpetrators of such humiliation will actually sit outside the shop at a window seat. They press the fart machine controller button and enjoy the surprise and mortifying "entertainment" inside—while innocently enjoying a cup of java outside. No lawsuits for invasion of privacy or for the intentional infliction of emotional distress have been recorded since the gag gift's invention. Even so, there is no question that not everyone is amused by remote control fart machine gags. Some consumers report that radio signals from other remote control devices will interfere and set off the electronic farts at inopportune times when the machines are being hidden. In these instances, the prankster gets pranked.

Remote control electronic fart machines are now in their second and third generation of development. The newer remotes for the devices reportedly can operate from longer distances. The machines have been miniaturized for placement under small pillows and chair cushions. Also, the new controllers allow for a broader scale of fart intonations. Selections can range from cheek squeakers to rip-ass farts with maximum auditory impact. Looking to the future, fart machine aficionados are yearning for the addition of olfactory circuitry contributions or smell accessories to accompany auditory effects. Such improvements are not out of the question. Any added "odorama" capabilities would presumably draw on technology from the days when cinemas experimented with Smell-O-Vision.[3] This was a system that released odor during a film's projection so that audiences could "smell" what was happening on the movie screen.

For those with a hankering for simpler, less high-tech fart devices, the Giant Yellow Fart Button is a novelty gift that offers funny noises with no nose pinching required. Realistic sound effects are produced by simply pressing a button to release the sound of bubbling flatulence. The Giant Yellow Fart Button is advertised as a high-quality, wacky stress reliever that is ideal as an office desk paperweight. The fun button is always reliable with clear, easy-to-hear sound clips. Totally portable, the device is made for dropping in backpacks, purses, or even suit coat pockets when on the go. When the time is right, the button can be pushed and some silly fun is activated. It's a modest machine, but IT offers a nice variety of farts, from tiny pips and putts to thrilling chili-induced trouser-tremblers.

An even simpler device for more elementary fart humor is the Fart Alarm Hand Bell. No assembly is required and no batteries are needed. This gag gift may be intended to send a message to the knaves who have taken far too much pleasure in offending others with their flatulence. The alarm bell is advertised as a dead ringer for clearing out ground zero when a particularly nasty guff is nigh—give the bell a few hard rings and everyone should get an unmistakable warning. A Fart Alarm Hand Bell is found to be particularly useful when employed in a bathroom to warn children and adults alike that there may be ample reason to avoid the room for a reasonable interval.

Kinder, Gentler Fart Toys

Kinder, gentler, quieter fart toys and gifts can include traditional stuffed animals. For more than a century, the teddy bear has comforted youngsters. The cuddly bear has a long history traced back to the presidency of Theodore Roosevelt. A 1904 political cartoon in *The Washington Post* inspired a toymaker to come up with the baby bear toy.[4] The original cartoon featured a frustrated Roosevelt with his rifle and a tiny black bear tied to a tree behind him. According to the legend, the American president refused to shoot the bear that was captured by his aides so that he could have a trophy like other hunters on an outdoor adventure.

In contrast to Roosevelt's sensitivity for the tiny growler and his reticence to harm the black bear, mothers may be tempted to shoot the farting teddy bear after hearing its refrains too many times, such as "I love you this much—'FART'—That was not me!" The farting teddy bear obviously is not as innocent as it looks, but at least the little fellow has enough shame to try to disown the indiscretions. The plush brown bear is advertised to please: "Hug its heart, to hear it fart." After given a squeeze, the bear offers a multitude of witty phrases topped off with hilarious farting sounds.

The playful teddy bear may be deemed too tame as a farting animal gag gift by hardcore flatulence enthusiasts. They may be much more disposed to investigate what the PlayMonster Stinky Pig has to offer. The Stinky Pig is an animated porker with a belly button that activates his singing and his other noise-making. Stinky Pig is advertised as a "fartastic" gift for the family because he can be the object of game nights for children together with their parents. When Stinky Pig's belly is pressed, he starts to sing a funny tune. Players must hurry up and roll the dice to see which way to pass Stinky Pig and do it quickly before he rips off a toot. Whoever is caught holding the pig when the oinker lets off a stinker must then take a token. The game is played until the token pile is gone and the player with the least number of tokens wins.

Parents can turn a vulgar and boorish game into an educational exercise by insisting that each player say, "Excuse me" when caught holding the farting bear. This game adaptation reinforces good manners for children and any child stuck with Stinky Pig is probably going to be less upset. The youngster is likely to enjoy the opportunity to ask to be pardoned after the pig does an inappropriate boom-boom.

If a fanny floater exiting from a Stinky Pig or a butt cough hacked from a teddy bear does not float the proverbial boat, then the solution for the discriminating flatulence lover may be something more presidential in nature. That would call for the Pull My Finger Farting Donald Trump Doll with Animated Hair. The Trump Doll emits the kind of greasy "wet farts" one might expect from any human being who devours quarter-pound patties from burger joints and buckets of fast-food chicken.

Farts from the ample posterior of the Donald John Trump Doll would not be particularly amusing on their own. However, several atomic burrito bonuses complete the presidential package. After one squeezes his index finger, the fart, of course, emerges strongly, very strongly. Then the signature orange hair lifts up high, thanks to the gassy breeze, and the orange top is actually in danger of leaving the premises.

The Trump Doll also delivers several phrases, including one blaming the gas emissions on Mexicans, the nationality that he has riffed on for years. Trump's other fine flatulence lines include "That fart was made in China," "That wasn't me, it was ISIS," and his boast "That's what I call a twoot. Trademarked." The vocals are amazingly close to Trump's actual voice and the attention to detail is spot-on. The doll is adorned with orange skin and white-rimmed eyes, a lengthy red necktie, and fluffy orange hair that takes "The Donald" to the next level for authenticity.

After palling around with The Donald, a president famous for years of consorting with well-coiffed, pulchritudinous women in Moscow nightclubs and Atlantic City beauty pageants, an appropriate perfume or cologne might be in order. And what cologne could be more appropriate for someone who appreciates the Pull My Finger Farting Donald Trump Doll than the Gagster No. 2 ASSence Prank Perfume Liquid Fart Spray Fragrance Gift Kit. Clever packaging for the ASSence brand of fart spray is one of the attractions that lures shoppers to purchase what looks to be a luxurious scent.

Even a short hit of the spray, however, reveals a fragrance described as the odor of an abandoned public toilet in a climate change heat wave or the aroma of a bloated skunk that ate a week-old meat lovers' pizza. Those who've had some acquaintance with ASSence advise a quick departure from the room in which it has been sprayed. This is because the raunchy smell can easily be categorized as a biohazard. For that reason, it is sometimes recommended that ASSence be sprayed out on a deck or back porch where it can be savored briefly, yet given the quick slip for sanity's sake.

Most fart-related gag gifts are of little practical value, though it can be argued that nothing is more practical in this world than the comfort of a good giggle or a laugh inspired by a fart gift. Nevertheless, all arguments to the contrary, there is nothing especially practical about a Fart Alarm Hand Bell or a Pull My Finger Farting Donald Trump Doll. One item that does have some practical value in the overflowing cornucopia of fart merchandise are Shart Wipes.

In the product description for Shart Wipes, this gift is classified as a "must-have for everyone"—and especially anyone who has owned a butt all their life. Most butt owners have been mortified at some point in their life by a rogue squirt or the green apple dirties. According to the product description, friends simply do not leave their friends unprepared without Shart Wipes. This is because nobody is exempt from nasty surprises. Everyone at some point is forced to do the "shameful backward walk" to the nearest bathroom to clean up an unexpected mess.

Shart Wipes to the Rescue

Shart Wipes come in handy for those who mistakenly believe that they can get away with a "silent but deadly" at church, school, the grocery store, the office, a PTA meeting, or a ladies' luncheon. When it turns out that there was a little more loaded in the cannon than expected, there can be a crisis. Most people have experienced an unwisely trusted fart in their life, much to their regret. That's when Shart Wipes can come to the rescue. They're the ideal size for concealment yet pack enough clean-up power to handle any situation when sharts happen. Shart Wipes are touted as truly awesome additions to all gift baskets, birthday presents, and Christmas stockings. In testimonials, Shart Wipes even get the nod of approval for placing in care packages to military personnel stationed overseas.

It's logical to ask: If Shart Wipes are on the fart gift short list for enlisted men, can a brand spanking new three-pack of Code Brown Commandos Emergency Underpants be far behind? The unique underwear comes packed in a small tin container, which allows them to be carried in a pants pocket inconspicuously and pulled out when an unexpected need arises. There are also one-use granny panties made of comfortable polyester fabric and designed to be super-stretchy, which means they can fit men and women, large or small.

The Commandos Emergency Underpants are best suited for the macho guy who's into guns and ammo, war games, and enemy ambushes—the kind of guy who insists on being prepared in case he has an "accident" in the field. These are definitely no-frills tighty-whities for the man who is less interested in making a fashion statement and more interested in plugging leaks that would give aid and comfort to all adversaries. In brief, these battle-ready undies provide the freedom to eat whatever tastes great in other lands, even if the eating experience never seems to come out well in the end.

Coffee, tea and other caffeine drinks frequently have a laxative potential that can lead to a bad case of the Hershey squirts—and the usual accompanying acoustics. The acidic nature of brewed beverages can prompt the body to produce more bile, the sort of bitter, alkaline substances that make stomachs churn. This in turn can cause a build-up in the gut causing a bad case of the runs. While there is no perfect antidote to caffeine-induced fecal incontinence, the best advice is to be on guard for excessively loose stools before sitting down on a coffee house stool. Habitual coffee drinkers would be well advised to keep a tin of Code Brown Commandos Emergency Underpants, along with an emergency pack of Shart Wipes, on any extended outing to Starbucks.

True friends of coffee drinkers would do well to provide their coffee connoisseur colleagues with special Shart Wipes, the emergency undies, and a thoughtful selection from the wide range of fart coffee mugs that are available. Before choosing the most appropriate fart java jug or just the right farting coffee mug, it makes sense to assess what kind of coffee drinker is destined to receive the drinking device.

In making a proper evaluation for a fart coffee mug gift purchase, there are some pertinent questions to consider: Is the coffee drinker downing that cup of joe for a morning rush and to boost alertness and productivity for office work? Is the coffee drinker leisurely consuming the caffeinated beverage to improve various aspects of brain health, such as memory, mood, awareness, and general cognitive function? Is the coffee drinker clasping that steaming cup of brew to stave off headache, fatigue, anxiety, irritability or depression? Is the coffee drinker primarily interested in boosting flatulence potential?

There are some other pertinent questions to ponder in making a fart coffee cup selection, especially if the criteria to be considered is less about the liquid and more about the flatus. For example, does the coffee drinker have a reputation for reveling in ripping off farts of seismic proportion? Is the coffee drinker the quiet, shy type and easily embarrassed and more likely to emit a squeaker or silent-but-deadly variety of fart?

Age also can be a factor in all of this. Starting at about age 60, men are often resigned to passing more gas in larger amounts and with noticeably more frequency.[5] A coffee mug emblazoned with derogatory sarcasm that pokes fun at those seniors prone to the "green apple dirties" can be downright hurtful. On the other hand, a mug that simply offers a light-hearted tease—about the "one-that-got-away" fart or the "funny chicken scream" fart—may just bring a big smile to grandpa's face.

Best Grandfarter Ever

To bring this fart coffee cup discussion to some closure, here is just a sampling of what's out there when it comes to sloganeering on a coffee cup regarding the topic of cutting the cheese: "I Didn't Fart ... My Butt Blew

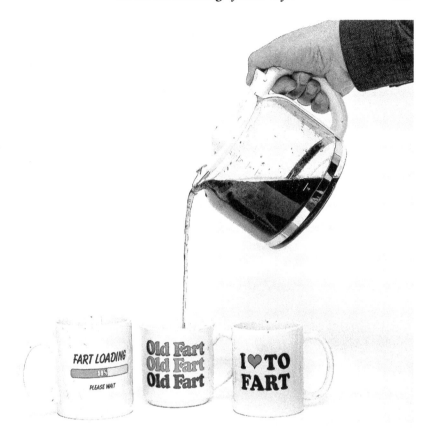

An endless number of fart souvenir mugs are given away to confirmed coffee drinkers at birthdays and during the holidays every year. Ironically, the caffeinated drinks can bring forth an unwanted bevy of farting (photograph by Ursula Ruhl).

You a Kiss," "Danger … Fart Machine," "Fart Loading … Please Wait," "Old Fart," "Best Grandfarter Ever," "I'm One Fart Away from a Poo," "Excuse Me but I Have to Fart," "Who Farted?" "World's Best Fart-Her," "Work Hard. Play Hard. Fart Hard," "F.A.Q. Fart and Quack," "Live. Fart. Laugh," "I Fart. What's Your Superpower?" "iFart," "I [Heart] to Fart," "Never Trust a Fart," "Powered by Unicorn Fartz," "I Don't Fart, I Just Whisper in My Pants," and "I Love Farting."

On the subject of fart coffee mugs, there are more and more mugs equipped with the oscillating electronic circuitry to provide bubbly farting noises while imbibing a brewed beverage. The novelty mugs are made of durable ceramic to withstand endless cups of coffee and jarring belly laughs. There is an on/off switch on the bottom of the mugs so the humor can be turned on and off at will. The mug also is dishwasher safe because the bottom of the electronic fart machine can be removed with a screwdriver and the mug placed in the dishwasher. Reading the side of the coffee cup is not required for these beaker squeakers, one can see—and hear—the coffee mugs actually speak for themselves. They can provide more than half a dozen fart sounds, ranging from short pop tarts to longer seam splitters and badger burps.

Fart socks, fart shorts, fart pants, fart shirts, fart slippers, and fart undergarments may not be electrified, but there's plenty of inert fart apparel available in cotton, polyester, spandex, rubber blends and more. With the "It's OK to Fart" stretch socks, there's a way to let the world know that one-cheek sneaks, puffers, squeakers, crop dusters, butt trumpets and turtle burps are no longer cause for shame. T-shirts, blouses and pullovers also carry the message that farting is a popular pastime for the impressive number of fart enthusiasts in North America. One of the most coveted tunics is an acronym-adorned, sleeveless shirt with the giant letters: DTF. The three print letters warn all those nearby that this jersey wearer has heart and is "Down to Fart"!

Flatulence quips and fart slogans from Hollywood movies are always in vogue on outerwear. The *Blazing Saddles* campfire farting T-shirt is a must on any camping trip where pork and beans are served. Of course, *South Park* must get into the act with a shirt sporting the words "You Fart Loving Tricksters! I'll Take Care of You!!!" The *Christmas Vacation* quote from Aunt Bethany, "Did I fart?" is always a hit when emblazoned on a shirt. It's especially cute when Aunt Bethany's hat and adorable face find a place on this holiday flatulence apparel.

CHAPTER 11

Farts

All About Male Bonding?

A distraught mother cries out in desperation about the problem of transporting young boys around in a van. They all insist on passing the most horrendous gas imaginable every time she is carpooling them. Noxious odors are released on the way home from school, or on the way to Scout meetings, or on the way to baseball diamonds at the athletic fields, and then on the rides back to their homes. All it takes is one young male to rip off a monster and soon there is relentless competition to match the original methane bomb. The sophomoric laughter is tolerable. The rude noises are disgusting. The trapped odor is intolerable. Will it damage the upholstery? Will it remain in the car seat foam forever?

The deeply depressed mother is beside herself and tired of sitting beside uncontrollable urchins that smell like a cross between a road-kill skunk and great globs of maggoty meat disintegrating in a garbage can at the height of summer heat. She is seriously offended, totally frustrated, tired of the joke, and completely uninterested in trying to "get" the joke. She wants to swear off motherhood, abandon the van in a grocery store parking lot, and take a normal-sized sedan on a road trip to anywhere—by herself. Perhaps she would consider driving off a Grand Canyon precipice with another mother named Thelma or Louise?

In "Farting, Fellowship, and Forgiveness," an article found on the *Man-Making Blog* by Earl "R.J." Cyler, the blogger argues that women have a more circumspect relationship with the part of the human experience known as flatulence.[1] As a consequence, they are very often offended by the attention focused on the passing of gas. Males, however, especially boys and adolescent dudes, have a more celebratory relationship with bodily functions involving methane. The phenomenon of taking pleasure in, or laughing at, the release of farts seems to be imprinted in the male DNA.

The *Man-Making Blog*, a self-described "practical and inspirational resource for people interested in supporting our young males on their

129

journey to manhood," cited another blog especially for moms that took up the issues of youthful male farting. A post on that blog noted the counter-productive exercise of a school giving detentions to a boy who caused a commotion by farting on the school bus. School authorities should under-stand that any punitive action levied on a young boy for flatulence is likely an exercise in futility.

One mom cited in the *Man-Making Blog* article received high praise for showing some "boy-literacy" when she said, "You know, I don't like anyone smelling up an enclosed space any more than the next gal, but fart-ing is practically an art form for a pre-teen boy." She also suggested that the young man, with his gaseous declaration of aspirational manhood, had "just bought himself a one-way ticket to popularity-ville."[2]

A deep dive into adolescent farting will reveal that the boy on the bus probably bought himself something more than a brief interlude of popu-larity. He was creating a memorable moment and also participating in the ancient ritual of male bonding. The creator of the *Man-Making Blog* postu-lated that the joys young males take in creative flatulence goes back to the activities of cave dwellers long before men were absorbed in watching tele-vised Super Bowls, spring college basketball playoffs or baseball's World Series.

Cave guys got their thrills by sitting around a fire, much as today's men sit around sports broadcasts on the wide screen. Cavemen relaxed after chowing down on a gargantuan meal of meaty mastodon or fresh venison and then let the digestive juices do their thing. As a little time passed, so did the gas. With very few social constraints, meat farts soon filled the living quarters of the cave dwellers. Inevitably, the noisy enter-tainment evolved into a competition accompanied by laughter, boasting, jealousy, and awe. Memories were made, bonds were forged, and the gas exhibitions undoubtedly reinforced the prominence and the dominance of the alpha males in the caveman pack.

Obviously, if there is something this ancient and enduring in the primal experience and make-up of the male gender, then it is probably a hopeless gesture for a school principal to discipline a farting boy or for a mother to insist on decorum in the carpool van. Birds gotta fly, girls gotta sing, boys gotta let their farts fly. It's gross and it's uncouth, and it's discouraged in polite society. However, when farting is outlawed, only outlaws will fart. And all boys are outlaws in this respect. And it's about something more than boys just being boys. Those farting cavemen of pri-mordial times are still very much with us.

A small helping of anecdotal experience, a bare modicum of human awareness, both combine to make it clear that flatulating adolescent boys do not all mature into men of propriety and decorum. More evolution is

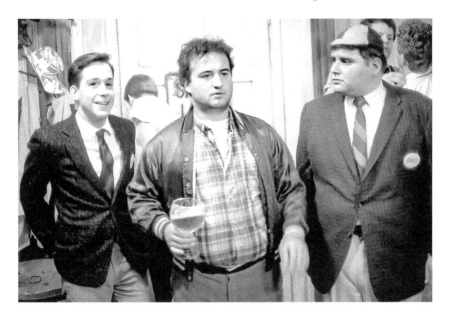

Drinking beer, cutting beer farts, and discussing flatulence have always been among the rituals that hold together the brotherhood of fraternity life. *National Lampoon's Animal House* (1978) featured the late John Belushi as Bluto (center) instructing a pledge, Kent "Flounder" Dorfman played by Stephen Furst (right), on fraternity etiquette. Also shown is Tom Hulce as Larry "Pinto" Kroger (Universal Pictures/Photofest).

required in so many instances. In his article "A Fine Bromance: The 12 Rules of Male Friendship," author Chris Moss concludes in his exploration of male bonding that flatulence is part and parcel of male relationships.[3] Successful male companionship is a delicate balance between altruism and selfishness with several dollops of flatulence mixed into a mysterious formula.

Moss concedes it would be more edifying to finish his listing of rules for male friendship with a quote from a male feminist or the philosopher Plato. Instead, he goes ape-like for one final rule in his otherwise distinguished essay about men being tribal—and he emphasizes that flatulence is an essential aspect of the tribalism. He argues that when four male PhDs are gathered together, or when six male gynecologists are assembled, or even when the 12 disciples broke bread at the Last Supper, it's always okay to break wind among friends.

"It is a taboo-prover, one of the things you generally don't do with acquaintances, work colleagues, women, children, but you can do it loudly, rudely, with mates," declares Moss. "This is tribal, animal, elemental—but it is also bathetic. The ability to lower the tone and make all the preceding chatter and thoughtfulness seem absurd and pretentious is itself a sort of philosophical position. There's nothing like an anti-climax for raising everyone's spirits."[4]

Scent of a Man Bonding

Sociologists claim that American men have always struggled to bond meaningfully with other males, to form serious or emotional relationships with other men. Men do find it easy to bond in superficial ways, whether that's in the form of sports entertainment, martial arts, the military, competitive games, or outdoor activities. Men will also bond in ways that confirm traditional male identity, such as partying and drinking together or just farting around in informal settings. However, not all men are passionately interested in these kinds of pursuits.

The rise of feminism in the 1970s through to the present has inspired the formation of various masculinist movements that are perhaps less visible than women's organizations. Men do increasingly yearn for deep, genuine connections with other men that don't depend on masculine norms like competitiveness, winning, dominance, violence, primacy of work, or pursuit of status. Contemporary masculinist movements are attracting males who ask such questions as: Is the traditional definition of masculinity obsolete? As the roles of women are changing in a new century, am I keeping up with how men's roles are changing? Amidst societal turmoil, can a man find refuge or safe haven in a men's group? Can I fart there?

Academics commonly identify eight major tendencies in what can be termed "the terrain of the politics of masculinities."[5] These tendencies shape the various categories of men's movements and can be summarized as follows: mythopoetic men's movement, the Promise Keepers, the Million Man Marchers, men's right advocates, men's liberationists, socialist feminist men, radical feminist men, and gay male liberationists. Some of these groups may be totally comfortable with a laissez-faire approach to farting while others may be inclined to put the lid on flatulence. Others may view the question of open expression of gas passing as beyond—or below—their purview.

The mythopoetic men's movement is associated with poet Robert Bly's 1990 book *Iron John*, which espouses inner discovery through tribal contact with other men.[6] The modus for discovering what makes men uniquely masculine can sometimes be all-male gatherings that include chanting, singing, drumming, and bonding encounters. When this movement gets publicity, it sometimes involves the media satirizing its process of discovery—the "wild man" ethic. This involves men gathering for intensive camping or tribal experiences. This group does not pose a threat to male farting and may actually encourage flatulence.

The Promise Keepers are a Christian men's movement that has been attacked from many quarters but particularly by women's groups and gay men's organizations. The Promise Keepers are religious traditionalists consistent with a biblical view that man has dominance over Earth, the fish and the fowl, and, of course, women.[7] Males are encouraged to acknowledge and atone for their mistakes in failing to support their wives, families, and communities. The Promise Keepers do not pose a threat to fundamental male perspectives on farting.

The Million Man Marchers are men of color who have been attracted to ideas about the family promulgated by Louis Farrakhan. Tagged as an extremist, Farrakhan has organized the marches for the Nation of Islam to position himself as a moderate or centrist.[8] As with the Promise Keepers, males are encouraged to acknowledge and atone for their failures to support their wives, families, and Black communities. Farting is not considered a character flaw and Million Man Marchers do not jeopardize traditional male perspectives on farting.

Men's right advocates are the most anti-feminist of all these masculinist organizations. Their views are reflected in such Warren Farrell books as *The Liberated Man* and *The Myth of Male Power*.[9] Feminism is viewed by these masculinists as a plot to cover up the reality that it is actually women who have all the power and men who are oppressed by current gender arrangements. Men's shorter life spans, health problems, and military conscription are all evidence that society favors women, according to men's right advocates. Farts are safe with these activists, but they contend that farting simply offers more fodder for women to nag men about their behavior.

Men's liberationists are modern males who tend to be professional and upper class. They are not necessarily angry with women who are feminists, but they do want permission to abandon the burdens of breadwinner status. Their basic platform is that both men and women have been oppressed by sexism.[10] They are interested in an intellectual approach to sex role theory and in broadening their own lifestyle choices. Freedom for farting at will (or at Wilhelmina) is not a given with this group. If women do not want males to fart in their presence, men should respect their wishes.

Socialist feminist men are primarily focused on equity issues. This group is focused on women's issues from an economic perspective and attempts to place them in the context of Marxist analysis of capitalist institutions. Many members of this group are academics who can be found on university campuses, very often in the faculty lounge, which is generally a fart-free zone. While farting may be frowned upon, it is not an important concern. In fact, farting may be a useful tool in general class struggle. The Bernie Sanders wing of socialist feminist men has some history of mobilizing flatulence in the service of protesting an oppressive and unresponsive system.

Radical feminist men probably pose the greatest threat to flatulence freedom, because the emission of male gas is viewed from the standpoint of toxic masculinity. Flatulence freedom is viewed as just a license to humiliate women, as one more weapon in the male arsenal to degrade women. Radical feminist men have been criticized for having a narrow focus on "male sexual violence" as a locus of men's oppression of women.[11] They also are sometimes dismissed as just an adjunct or a subsidiary of the feminist movement.

Gay male liberationists are not necessarily fart averse, but they are adamantly opposed to demeaning gay fart jokes. Their primary mission is to ensure for gay men the same status, rights, and privileges accorded to those in the "straight world."[12] In other words, gay male liberationists are more focused on efforts to achieve rights for the sexually diverse rather than on promoting any particular cultural agenda. Men in this group are neither for nor against flatulence freedom. They simply view the issue as a distraction and a rabbit hole that they have no interest in going down.

All these men's movement advocates have searched for points of agreement on social and cultural issues or just "common ground" that could bring together the various strands of an assortment of specialized interests. The thought is that focusing on points of agreement could help build coalitions that would make the men's movement more effective in the political area. However, it's fairly obvious that there is no real consensus on flatulence freedom among the diverse factions.

There is no inclination among these groups, with a few exceptions, to view flatulence as an appropriate catalyst for male bonding. Male bonding has to be about much more than the sulfuric aroma of a shared cloud of flatulence. Traditional males are likely to dismiss this stance as the result of over-thinking the issue. Real men don't need a men's movement in their view. And they certainly don't need academic symposia to decide the question of whether to fart or not to fart or whether farting is a means for men to bond together—that's just an unconscious given.

Farts, Sports, and Armed Forces

In sports and in the military, two familiar refuges for the traditional male, there is a reverence for the art of flatulence and for its time-worn role in the phenomena of male bonding. In the sports locker room, there is the ritual of crop dusting the entire team with the unmistakable fragrance of strategic flatulence. Crop duster farts are the aromatic glue that can hold a team together or that can cement the mission of a military platoon or company.

For the uninitiated, a crop duster fart involves the act of moving while passing gas, usually silently, thereby "dusting" other people in a confined area with acrid intestinal gas. Crop dusters are sometimes used to conceal the identity of the emission originator. The perpetrator tries to deliver the goods on the run. Crop dusting locations for this kind of subterfuge can include a supermarket, which can involve a quick stroll down the produce aisle, or it can involve inconspicuous browsing in the seafood section to break some wind to be purposely lost amidst competing odors.

In sports or in military venues, the goal for a crop duster is to make an impression on as many of the assembled as possible and also to be ready to take immediate ownership if a heavy dusting has the desired effect. That desired effect is to have as many peers as possible moaning in anguish and seeking cover. The act of crop dusting is a close kin to the act of carpet bombing, although a crop duster is generally of the "silent-but-deadly" variety of flatulence. Carpet bombing is noisy and meant to inspire terror even before the aromatic gas delivery is detected.

Crop dusting is a team sport, but the ultimate fart for male-bonding purposes is a mano-a-mano affair. There may be no more sacred rite of passage in the cult of flatulence bonding than the act of farting directly on a friend. It's a practice that has been passed down from generation to generation, father to son, sometimes from crazy old uncle to innocent, visiting nephew. There's really nothing equal for showing one male that another male sincerely cares for him than to intimately deliver a fart of substance.

In a post on the blog site *A Beast, an Angel, and a Madman*, Albert Riehle recalls the story from 2005 when the Chicago Cubs traded pitcher Greg Maddux and closer Ryan Dempster, who shared so much together in the locker room, including their flatulence.

"We've been sharing locker space for three years," Dempster said. "It's kind of weird not having him there to talk about golf or about pitching, farting on each other...."[13]

Blogger Riehle noted that the parting and the loss of friendship farting had to bring such sadness: "I remember feeling bad for Ryan Dempster, the author of the above quote," observed Riehle in his 2007 post. "He will never again come back to the locker after a particularly rough game, when he gave up a game winning home run to some guy from the other team, the weight of a loss on his shoulders, frustration brimming inside him, only to be farted on by Greg Maddux making everything, somehow all right."

"And so I say to you, enjoy your friend's farts while you have them men," declared Riehle. "You never know when they'll be taken away from you, or traded to the Dodgers."[14]

In the male-bonding ritual that involves flatulence, Riehle insists that it is incumbent upon the man expressing his affection to be able to produce farts of glorious magnitude. Likewise, a friend on the receiving end must put aside any individual bravado and bask in the gas with appropriate humility—while the farter sits back and enjoys the glory and triumph of his noxious fumes.

Riehle continues: "I think about my own friends and how we may be sitting around when all of the sudden one of them not only rips one, but feels the need to fan it in my general direction, spreading the wealth, if you will. Is he trying to make my eyes water? Sure. Is he trying to make me gag? Of course. But the underlying message in that fart, the true purpose of it is to say, 'Hey.... I love you man!'"[15]

The male-bonding ritual of professional baseball athletes like Greg Maddux and Ryan Dempster is, of course, shared by many of the grunts in the U.S. military. Athletes and soldiers share what appears to be a mainstay of male-bonding culture in America. Unfortunately, foreign nationals do not always share, understand, or sympathize with this somewhat peculiar and pungent aspect of American culture. This can mean trouble. Ann Jones, author of the book *Kabul in Winter: Life Without Peace in Afghanistan*, wrote about cultural misunderstanding in America's longest war in 2010.

Jones explained in her war reporting for the *TomDispatch.com* that American soldiers were losing the hearts and minds of their Afghan allies in the war against the Taliban because of their excessive farting. Young American soldiers were alienating many of their would-be supporters in Afghanistan with their locker-room-style, male-bonding bouts of hilarious farting.

In her dispatch titled "Ugly Americans Farting Their Way to Alienation," Jones explained the perspective of men in Afghanistan toward the American obsession with farting: "To Afghan men, nothing is more shameful. A fart is proof that a man cannot control any of his apparatus below the belt. The man who farts is thus not a man at all. He cannot be taken seriously, nor can any of his ideas or promises or plans."[16]

The Afghan men serving as interpreters for U.S. soldiers were reportedly embarrassed to the point of agony over the American male farting. They were desperate to put a stop to it. The U.S. military made effort after effort to meet and make friends with village elders, drink tea, plan "development" for the country's future. Several interpreters told Jones that every meeting was sabotaged by a bevy of young American soldiers breaking wind without regard to cultural norms in Afghanistan.

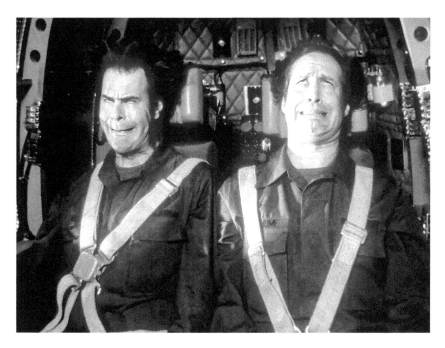

Dan Aykroyd (left) and Chevy Chase play two hapless special agents in *Spies Like Us* (1985). Flatulence is an important part of male bonding in fraternity houses, in sports locker rooms, in military barracks, and in special intelligence operations. Chevy Chase breaks most of the wind in *Spies Like Us* (Warner Bros./Photofest).

At first unaware of these occurrences, the U.S. Army simply went on with its meetings and planning efforts to build infrastructure, to promote good governance, and to generally "do good" in Afghanistan to counter a primitive Taliban enemy. Eventually, awareness of the flatulence problems made their way up the command structure and U.S. authorities banned audible farting among the troops downrange. The justification was farting's counterproductive nature in the Afghan war effort.

The military's new rules in Afghanistan were reported by Gina Cavallaro in August 2011 in the *BattleRattle* magazine blog. She apologized for the story and advised readers that farts were not her beat. She did not want to report on the brass's order for soldiers not to fart when stationed in Afghanistan because it was offensive to the locals. She said there are many things the soldiers have had to give up because they are supposed to accommodate Afghan cultural norms.

Cavallaro wrote: "They're not supposed to cuss because it could be misunderstood (that one goes out the window a lot). And they stay away from talking about politics, religion or girls because those topics could escalate into major disagreements (they can't communicate anyway because of the language barrier)."

"But farting?" she continued. "That's practically a sport. OK, it's not soccer, but a good contest could open the door for cross-cultural exchanges, jokes and other gallows humor. So, for all Marines getting ready to go downwind, I mean downrange, be forewarned—you may have to hold it in … at least until you get back to your hooch where you can loudly crop dust your friends."[17]

Among the typical responses from America's warriors to Cavallaro's report on the military's fart ban in Afghanistan:

- "We are protecting them assholes. Boys, let 'em rip!"
- "I have to ask … what disciplinary action does UAF (Un-Approved Farting) carry these days?"
- "Oh … my … word…. Time to come home, boys, lest we offend the delicate sensibilities of those gentle Afghans."
- "Next thing they're gonna do is take away throwing rocks, talkin' about our women, sharing poop stories, and the rest of the things Marines do when we have nothing else besides waiting to wait. General, sir, I am disinclined to aquester your request. Semper Fidelis, Yat-Yas…."
- "If we can't fart around the Afghans, then they should stop wiping their fecal matter all over the port-o-potties. Fair trade."
- "I think its sorta funny that Afghanis can go and take a dump on the side of the road or get it on with a goat in their front yard but passing gas is offensive. Really? Who gives a … flying fart what they think?"
- "Farting is a key morale builder. The act of having a compatriot yank your finger in order to release a fart is as ancient a practice as when Alexander crossed the Kush."
- "During my time in the service, farting as loudly and poisonously as possible was looked on with high esteem. Now, we have to actually restrain a natural part of our biology because of the hypersensitivity of some people in a turd world country? Good grief!"

In August of 2021, America's longest war ended when Afghanistan fell to the Taliban. The departure of Americans from the airport in Kabul was ignominious at best. Afghan troops who were allies of the Americans against the Taliban folded in a matter of days when it became clear American troops and advisers were leaving. Their surrender to the Taliban has raised many questions about what the war effort was all about, how much blood and treasure were lost over two decades, and why the war effort failed. To date, however, no one is asking what role American male flatulence played in the collapse of our U.S. allies in Afghanistan.

CHAPTER 12

Farting Goddesses
Air Grievances

Women have long been put on a pedestal and their bodies shown off like statuesque, porcelain figures of perfection. Their female bodies never grow tired; they do not put on weight; they do not leak; they do not give off odors; they do not make unexpected noises—they certainly do not fart. Women on the pedestal are envied and emulated by their less attractive and lower status sisters. These women on the pedestal are idealized, desired, and worshipped by men. These women of stature stand apart, but they share an ancient lineage. They are the descendants of goddesses with classic names like Venus, like Isis, like Luna, like Flora.

As the goddess of love, Venus is one of the most famous and most important goddesses. Venus is usually represented as a nude, stunning, voluptuous woman. Isis is a celestial goddess who is associated with a beautiful full moon, and she has admirers sighing to the heavens. Luna also has a special relationship with the moon. Luna is most often pictured as a beautiful woman with a moon crescent adorning her head, worn as a sort of tiara. Flora is the ancient goddess of flowers and edible plants. She is usually portrayed as a beautiful woman carrying flowers in her hands.

The goddesses are beautiful and much admired, but they are tired of suppressing their gas. If men can fart selfishly and impose their male toxic gas on loved ones, then why should a goddess have to restrain her flatulence? Venus wants to fart. Isis wants to fart. Luna wants to fart. Flora wants to fart. So does Fortuna, Diana, Bellona, Bona Dia, and Victoria. What happened to inspire this yearning among goddesses? With the rise of feminism in the 1970s, many goddesses—and women generally—let it be known that they want to climb down from their exalted perches. They want to smash their pedestals, which have alternately elevated them and at the same time caused them much anguish.

Goddesses—and women generally—are saying they're fed up with having to be "ladylike" at the behest of their male acquaintances. Female bodies don't just exist to be gazed upon by men—they can spring leaks; they do give off interesting odors; they are certainly capable of unexpected noises—and it is time for men "to just deal." Today's goddesses note that when their farts are suppressed, they suffer abdominally, sometimes with excruciating pain. What's more, suppressed gas can emerge as bad breath. In any case, not a single man is worth the gastrointestinal discomfort of women in the new millennium—girls, let 'em rip!

Men who take pride in the odor quotient of their own productions need to wake up and smell ... the coffee? Gastroenterologists point out that women's farts actually smell worse than

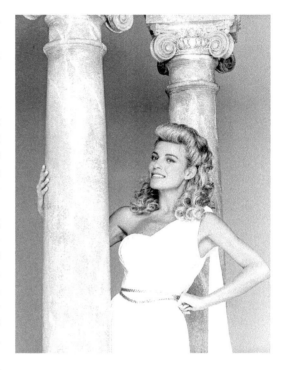

Women have always had difficulty living up to goddess standards—rules which allow for only a bare minimum of flatulence. In the 1988 made-for-television movie *Goddess of Love*, a tight-cheeked Venus, played by Vanna White, comes to Earth to find love with guidelines from Zeus (NBC/Photofest).

men's, according to many scientific studies.[1] Also, some women actually have higher production rates for gas, though they surely are not as noisy or as proud of their flatulence as men. However, that situation could change as women become more comfortable with letting them rip.

Many fragile male egos—and their natural whoopee cushions—are likely deflating with the new knowledge that the flatulence given off by the opposite sex can be extremely pungent and often will smell worse than anything a man can produce. Scientists like gastroenterologist Michael D. Levitt, the author of scores of scholarly papers on the problem of intestinal gas, has confirmed that women's farts have far higher concentrations of hydrogen sulfide.[2] Hydrogen sulfide is a key ingredient in the smell factor of farts, along with methane, carbon dioxide, and other gases given off by specific bacteria in the intestinal track.

One of the most famous studies to clear the air on many feminine farting issues is that of L.G. Lippman titled "Toward a Social Psychology of Flatulence: The Interpersonal Regulation of Natural Gas," which appeared in a 1980 issue of *Psychology: A Quarterly Journal of Human Behavior.*[3] Lippman and others can confirm that women's farts are more odoriferous than the male variety. Men who take great pride in their flatulence can take some solace upon learning that the volume of rectal gas in a female fart is usually about 20 percent less than that of a male. Also, women tend to release a slightly smaller number of farts than men.

Regardless of the strength, number, and volume of farts passed by either gender on a daily basis, the inhaling spectators of all this rectal release can rest assured that flatulence is not unhealthy to breathe. Farting in the presence of others can be gross, uncouth, and disturbing, but it is not dangerous to physical health. However, the mental stress caused by flatulent companions can be another matter entirely.

Farting throughout the day and night is considered normal and a good thing health-wise by most experts who've studied the phenomenon. Flatulence is a natural occurrence and the by-product of a healthy digestive system at work. The body produces gas as part of breaking down and processing foods as a part of digestion. Monitoring the frequency and smell of farts is not a bad idea. Along with other gastrointestinal symptoms, they can be an indication of some potentially serious conditions. Goddesses are not immune.

Unfortunately, women who are predisposed to hold on to their gas, because that is the lady-like thing to do, are not just setting themselves up for uncomfortable bloating. Holding in intestinal gas can cause it to be reabsorbed into the bloodstream. It can then emerge as bad breath, which can be consistently offensive as compared to the transitory nature of a toot. Farting can be the lesser of two evil olfactory offenses and it definitely causes less discomfort.

End All Fart Shaming

Women have repeatedly complained about men who fart selfishly and impose their male toxicity on the very people they claim to love. What's even worse is the double standard when a woman is "fart-shamed" for inadvertently peeling off a squeaker on a couch or the living room easy chair. In the latest skirmishes in America's gender wars, more and more women are firing off some nasty volleys and then telling any offended men to go take a hike.

In earlier times, women went to ridiculous extremes to camouflage or cover up their rectal gas expulsions when out in public settings. Ladies of high society were known to take their faithful lap dogs with them everywhere. When they took tea in the parlor at a neighboring mansion, a woman's best friend would dutifully climb onto their laps as they settled in their chairs with some caffeinated drinks and scones. These women of refinement recognized the great benefit of being able to blame the dog when a foul smell sullied the parlor.

The scapegoated canines had to be specially trained to take the rap when on the old lady's lap. That's because dogs have a keen sense of smell and are much more sensitive to human farting than actual humans. They can react adversely to intense smells. Both dogs and humans are capable of putting out noxious fumes, especially of the meat-fart variety. That explains why pooches have been excellent patsies for taking the blame for some female flatulence in a dining room or anteroom. This may also explain why the ladies are gaga and so appreciative of the canines in the Westminster Dog Show.

Dogs really can be responsible for stinking up the place as any hound dog lover or veteran puppy owner can attest. This has been particularly true for hunting dogs that are regularly fed horse meat. Dogs obviously are natural chumps for taking the heat for an unwholesome gas releases by humans. A woman with a lap dog today can establish a perfect alibi after pooting in polite company in the parlor. She can give Rover a reproachful look and claim her own innocence by exclaiming: "Oh, Rover, I must have forgotten to give you your No Toot chews this morning." NaturVet sells No Toot Gas Aid for canines to address their wall clouds.

Of course, the Thoroughly Modern Millies of today have no need to drag around a pathetic lap dog to take the rap for their gas, nor do they need any ready alibis for their slippage. What's more, they also should have the confidence to tell men where to stick it, if rude males insist on shaming them after an accidental butt burp. A 2014 article by "Glosswitch" in *The New Statesman* makes this point on behalf of all women who have ever been fart-shamed.[4]

The New Statesman piece, titled "Why Farting Is a Feminist Issue," slams the unfairness of male privilege and the past double standard on passing gas: "A female body remains a thing to use, to own and to look at. It's not something which does things suggestive of some real, human messiness inside…. In contrast to the female body, the male body is simply allowed to *be*: to fill the room, legs spread wide, adding its own sounds and scents to the air. To assume the right to be a little bit revolting—to spit on the street, to jokingly raise your arse cheek to fart—is, I would argue, a form of privilege. It expresses an ownership not just of the body, but of the space around it."[5]

Although *The New Statesman* does not argue for feminist "Fart-In" demonstrations, it does argue for the right of women to occasionally raise an arse cheek to fart proudly. The era of the double standard is over. Feminists now maintain that any guy who tries to "fart-shame" his lady—after she exercises her natural right to express what she feels in her gut—must be dumped. The clarion call for women in the new millennium is simple: Dump the chump who tries to control your rump.

One sure sign that things are changing for women with flatulence in 2022 was the big news that a reality TV star was selling her farts in jars and making thousands of dollars. Stephanie Matto entered the personal gas business after rising to fame on the *90 Day Fiancé* TV show.[6] The self-described "fartrepreneur" ran into a buzz saw when she found out she could not keep up with demand. She was producing about 50 jars a week, but her level of output soon was not cutting it.

Matto apparently decided to change her diet to meet business demands, according to *Jam Press*.[7] She took on an expanded high-fiber diet with plenty of beans and eggs. Matto added protein shakes when she found that her farts smelled especially strong after adding the shakes to the mix. However, when the new diet began causing her excessive stomach pain, Matto knew she was getting so far behind with filling jars that something had to give, but not her. A visit to the hospital was such an unsettling experience, she finally realized it was time to back off from her ambitions as a fartrepreneur.

Matto may not have cut the mustard as the nation's first full-time, female fartrepreneur, but she had a message for the nation in that bottle. Women were no longer interested in the lifetime constraints of being lady-like. They no longer felt compelled to have a lap dog take the rap for a flatulence binge. Women were saying no to bottling up their gas, unless it was in an attractive dispensary bottle with a price tag attached.

What Do Women Want?

With the rise of the feminist movement, thousands of books have been written about their present milieu. What do women really want from life? What should women demand out of life? Most are probably not so interested in becoming "fartrepreneurs." Mainstream bookstores offer countless titles covering women's longings for romantic partners who can offer sensitivity, satisfying intimacy, and basic honesty. These books cover women's yearnings for higher levels of maturity, humility and trustworthiness from men. Books cover how women want regular offerings of kindness, patience, understanding, empathy, and compassion.

Some of the new books on women focus less on emotional needs and more on the practical support that they wish their partners could provide, which can mean being able to assist in both small and big ways, whether it's taking time to listen and to be more understanding or to be more active in decision-making, child-rearing, and finances. Women seek a positive and supportive presence. Women are less interested in brute strength and more interested in intelligence from a partner, according to women's book authors.

However, none of the many women's books cover what women really want in a relationship when it comes to flatulence. What explains that void? There are many questions to address when examining issues of flatulence in modern relationships. Some of these matters already have been touched upon in this study, but it is useful to take another look and also to summarize important findings in the recent gender flatulence debate. Some key points:

- Women say they don't want to be put on pedestals as goddesses with unrealistic expectations placed upon them. Accept that they are just human beings who occasionally have flatulence. So don't make a big deal about it when a freaky squeaker female fart takes the mainstage. A true gentleman abides by an unwritten rule which holds that if a lady does happen to break wind, he will turn a deaf ear to it. Under no circumstances does a gentleman try to get a woman to concede that she is responsible for escaping gas even when the auditory or olfactory evidence is beyond dispute. At the same time, if a woman takes ownership of a bit of flatulence, there is no need to congratulate her for being "one of the boys."
- Women say they don't appreciate fart gifts at Valentine's Day or for the children at Christmas or Hannukah. Any woman who has experienced a bout or two with excessive flatulence in her lifetime does not want a gift that provides some remembrance of farts past. Fart bags, whoopee cushions or "Fart Loading" coffee mugs are absolutely off the table. And a nice holiday can be totally ruined by children receiving fart gifts. Children have a tendency to play the audio on the farting teddy bear over and over again. Fathers may enjoy hearing their kids play the "Flight of the Buttock Bees" music on a battery-powered fart machine, but for mothers, the batteries will never wear down fast enough.
- Women say they are not interested in acquiring a vast vocabulary of fart synonyms and they are not impressed by men who can define and use such terms as bark, beef, bugle, backfire, break a tater, or burn bad powder. Having 500 vulgar words for breaking

wind at the ready is not a substitute for refinement. Using Old English or Latin terms for crackling noises that emanate from the back end does not indicate any kind of sophistication. For example, "crepitate" is used by a few sophists who are uncomfortable using the synonym "to fart." Peter Furze says as much in his book *Tailwinds: The Lore and Language of Fizzles, Farts and Toots.* Furze observes: "Crepitate was in occasional literary use in the seventeenth century, but was never a colloquial term. It is unlikely that the Elizabethans ever asked one another: 'Who crepitated?'"[8]

- Women say they don't want to be engaged in a "bromance" with a man. They do not want to be participants in the kind of antics described as male bonding exercises, such as farting on your best friend in the barracks or on your sports buddy in the locker room. That means no "Dutch ovens" in the boudoir. Men can foolishly think their relationship with a woman has cured or matured when they can fart in bed and force their partner's head under the sheets in order to appreciate the prolonged smell of a recently departed fart. A mattress flatulator should never assume a partner wishes to partake in the infamous Dutch oven and should exercise the courtesy of backfiring in the opposite direction of a bed partner.

We do admittedly live in a time of 50 shades of gray when not all the rules are in black and white—and some rules are made to be broken. Most women are not into S&M farting games. However, if a woman does say she wants to experiment with eproctophilia, her partner could be in for a wild ride. Fart fetishes do exist. There are individuals who derive sexual pleasure from rather strange smells and odors. Oddly enough, flatulence can be a turn on for some—and may constitute one of the newest shades in 51 shades of gray. However, flatulence experimentation should have mutual consent spelled out in black and white.

- Women say they do want to please their partners, but there are limits. Back in the 1960s' heydays of sex, drugs and rock 'n' roll, young men were studious readers of the liberating fiction of Philip Roth's *Portnoy's Complaint.* They read about kissing the bubbles: "When I fart in the bathtub, she kneels naked on the tile floor, leans all the way over, and kisses the bubbles."[9] If natural, homemade, organic bubbles are sweet enough for a woman's lips, then they must surely be good for a man's. When a man asks a woman to kiss the bubbles, then he better be ready to reciprocate. He needs to remember that hers will be smellier thanks to that goodly portion of hydrogen sulfide.

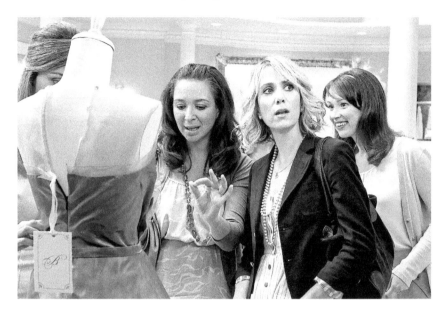

The 2011 comedy *Bridesmaids* shattered any illusions of women as goddesses holding in their belching, farting, snorting, or breaking wind. A bathroom debacle at the bridal shop, where the young women try on gowns, ranks among the movie industry's grossest bodily-function scenes. Shown from left are Maya Rudolph, Kristen Wiig, and Ellie Kemper (Universal Studios/Photofest).

Flatulence in relationships is all about trust and honesty. Fart enough to show humanity and vulnerability, but not so much as to drive a partner out of the room. As the self-professed "Fart Defender," Tracy Moore, declares: "Relationships start equally enough in fart terms, beginning in a fart-free zone of mutually understood politeness, an agreed-upon shielding of the other from your various emissions. But this should gradually give way to fart freely, at long last, together. When relationships become open season on bodily functions, they become more intimate. The couple who farts together stays together." Moore believes a couple must journey together to find their fart sweet spot.[10]

Feminists on Farts

Radical feminists and anti-porn feminists would have zero patience with Fart Defender Tracy Moore talking about women and men looking for the "fart sweet spot" together. Movement feminists take a dim view of whatever the patriarchy has to offer when it comes to bodily functions and the use of various human orifices. The patriarchy is not to be trusted. The previous chapter of this study surveyed the various subsets of the men's movement and how each male group is likely to position itself on flatulence issues. That kind of survey is not so easily accomplished with the women's movement.

The reason flatulence analysis is a far more daunting task in surveying the different subsets of feminism is because there are so many of them. First, consider that the feminist movement has encompassed four distinct "waves" of feminism, beginning with the cause of suffrage. Second, there are many articulations of feminism by many different names, such as radical feminism, separatist feminism, sex-positive feminism, anti-porn feminism, anarchist feminism, socialist feminism, eco-feminism, post-modern feminism, trans feminism, existential feminism, and, in recent times, punk or riot "grrls" feminism.

A simplified approach is to divide up the many factions and place them under two major headings of anti-porn feminism and pro-sex feminism. This may be where the rubber meets the road in getting a handle on feminist perspectives on flatulence. These two categories are clearly at odds with each other and they provide the starkest of contrasts. Anti-porn feminists arose in the late 1970s and found expression in the works of Andrea Dworkin, Catharine MacKinnon and Robin Morgan. Pro-sex, sometimes called sex-positive feminism, arrived about a decade later and was articulated by thought leaders such as Betty Dodson, Ellen Willis, and Gayle Rubin.

Anti-porn feminists Morgan and MacKinnon held that overtly sexual portrayals of women might be summarized as "pornography is the theory, rape is the practice." Heterosexual intercourse as exhibited in pornography is the essence of male domination. It must be banished because it is irredeemably harmful to women. Also, the porn industry has transformed sex into a packaged product. This has led to the further commodification and objectification of women. A central tenet of the anti-porn feminists is that ending pornography is essential for female liberation.

Pro-sex feminists take the view that pornography and the sex industry can actually be a source of empowerment and is not always degrading. Pro-sex feminists are libertarian and oppose legal or social efforts to control sexual expression between consenting adults, which can include watching pornography. Pro-sex feminists feel that anti-porn feminists too often vilify men and are simply anti-male. They also contend that feminists should avoid attacking other women's sexual proclivities and stop dismissing them as internalizing male oppression, or as kinky and unnatural, or as being just another impediment for the liberation of women.

Obviously, sex-positive feminists are going to be more open to "kink" and the idea of "fart games" in lovemaking. When they argue that sex is a natural force that precedes cultural life and institutional norms, they mean that flatulence is a similar force of nature—a powerful force of nature that can be reckoned with but not suppressed. For sex-positive feminists, it's all about the importance of consent when it comes to fart games. Consent is the process of setting boundaries, defining terms, and insisting on transparency and protection from harm. In simpler terms, if a man is going to put a woman in a meat-fart Dutch oven, he better know that his lady is all good for that and that he may have to be prepared for a little hydrogen sulfide release on her end.

In contrast to the sex-positive feminists, anti-porn feminists are not going to have much tolerance for "fart games" in the boudoir, or in the parlor sitting room, or anywhere else. The liberation of women must be understood within the historical framework of patriarchal domination and a chauvinism that is in some manner perfectly encapsulated in aggressive farting by men. True sexual liberation involves hard work and can only be achieved with an appreciation of the historic imbalance of power between men and women. In simpler terms, any woman who believes that she can reform some of the toxic, fetish-like, flatulence impulses of the male gender is in for a whole lot of anguish, mistaken intimacy, and inevitable disillusionment.

CHAPTER 13

Protest Farts

We Shall Not Be Moved

Farts have been a form of social protest—and a means of insulting and challenging authority—for centuries. In the age of kings and queens, subjects who farted in the presence of royalty were sometimes beheaded or hanged themselves out of shame and desperation. In more recent times, aggressive male farting aimed at females has been interpreted as a protest against feminism and the matriarchy. Such male farting has been denounced by some feminists as a demonstration of toxic masculinity meant to belittle women.

Protest farts also have been employed in demonstrations on issues ranging from gun violence to the need for minimum wage hikes at fast food restaurants. At the University of Texas in 2015, students used "mass farting" to protest mass shootings as well as the omnipresent gun culture in the Lone Star State.[1] In 2016, Bernie Sanders supporters organized a "fart-in protest" against Hillary Clinton meant to dramatize an "illusion of democracy" that they said was perpetuated by the Clinton campaign and the Democratic Party.[2] Fart-in demonstrations have taken place around the world but are especially notable in protest actions in the United States.

Fart-in demonstrations in the United States had their origin with the ultimate radical community organizer Saul Alinsky. The Chicago–based political theorist worked through the Industrial Areas Foundation to assist poor communities in organizing protest actions against landlords, elected officials, and business leaders. His leadership won him national recognition and his 1971 book *Rules for Radicals* may have given him eternal notoriety.[3] He died in 1972.

Alinsky was the father of the art of the "fart-in," a demonstration tactic which he threatened to unleash while organizing in Rochester, New York, to break Eastman Kodak's hold on what was essentially a company town. In a 1972 interview with *Playboy* magazine, Alinsky was asked whether a fart-in was not a bit juvenile and absurd. Alinsky replied that much of life is absurd, but the important thing was that the threatened demonstration at the Rochester symphony won concessions from Eastman Kodak.

He made four major points about the planned fart-in. First, the fart-in would take city officials totally by surprise. Demonstrations and picketing they could handle, but never in their wildest dreams could they envision a "flatulent blitzkrieg" inside the hall of their city's sacred symphony orchestra. The thought of a fart-in at their treasured musical sanctum threw them into complete disarray.

Second, the action would make a mockery of the law, because although you could be arrested for throwing a stink bomb, there's no law on the books against natural body functions like releasing farts at a symphony. Cops are known to take a favorable stance on farting and generally value a sweet fart as much as a glazed donut. The cops would be reluctant to arrest participants on charges of first-degree farting.

Third, when the news got around, everybody who heard it would break out laughing, and the Rochester Philharmonic and the establishment would be rendered ridiculous. Establishment types prefer to be looked upon as oppressive rather than ridiculous. A demonstration that holds authorities up to ridicule with non-violent tactics is far more effective than an unruly protest which threatens public safety and can inspire a backlash.

A fourth benefit of the tactic, according to Alinsky, was that it was psychically as well as physically satisfying to the demonstrators. "What oppressed person doesn't want, literally or figuratively, to shit on his oppressors?" asked Alinsky. "Here was the closest chance they'd have. Such tactics aren't just cute; they can be useful in driving your opponent up the wall. Very often the most ridiculous tactic can prove the most effective."[4]

In retrospect, not everybody was amused by the community organizer's tactics, including some Blacks who benefited from the Alinsky's fart-in threat. In an essay titled "So the Last Shall Be First...: Alinsky's Farting Negroes," Irmin Vinson contends that Alinsky's idea of organizing oppressed Blacks for a fart-in was condescending and implicitly racist. The declared political aims of Alinsky's proposed fart-in were to prompt Eastman Kodak to hire Blacks and to recognize the Black community's designated spokespersons. Vinson questions whether either of those objectives would have been realized by an actual fart-in.

Vinson writes: "On its face a hundred farting Blacks degrading themselves at a performance of the Rochester Philharmonic would have been an argument *against* hiring Blacks and *against* taking seriously any suggestions that their spokesmen might make. At the very least it would have made Blacks appear low and vulgar, leaving an impression which a genuine pro–Black activist would hope to avoid."[5]

Vinson also takes umbrage with an underlying assumption in Alinsky's plan that Blacks had some kind of immunity to the insufferable odors of a mass fart-in. Alinsky evidently assumed that the more refined and cultured a population, the more likely its members are to be distressed by a "flatulent blitzkrieg" in their sacred space. During the fart-in, cultured Caucasians who enjoyed symphonies would endure more than uncultured Blacks who knew nothing of symphony music. The low-status Blacks could defeat cultured Caucasians by their greater ability to tolerate the foul odors of passed gas.

An additional fantasy, according to Vinson, can be likened to a Marx Brothers' comedy. The Black protesters eat vast amounts of beans to weaponize themselves for the symphony. When they take their ticketed seats, they begin their own "symphony" to coincide with the orchestra's performance. Alinsky envisioned Rochester's high society ladies, a day after their precious symphony event had been convulsed by farting Black people, demanding of their husbands: "We are not going to have our symphony season ruined by *those people*! I don't know what they want but whatever it is, something has got to be done and this kind of thing has to be stopped!"[6]

Alinsky's confidence in the lowness of Blacks, according to Vinson, is entirely at odds with the movement during the last century for "positive negritude," which has as its goal the discrediting of the binary opposition that contrasts the civilization of Europeans to the savagery and non-civilization of Africans. Had the fart-in actually occurred, Vinson said it would not have been an example of the American Negro proclaiming himself in pride as Black, face-to-face with whites. Instead it would have been, to put it simply, an example of an angry Jewish organizer enlisting Blacks to degrade themselves for the purpose of attacking and offending the establishment and his own racial enemies.

Perhaps Vinson is over-thinking all the implications of Alinsky's planned fart-in. Perhaps Alinksy was engaging in grandiosity and overestimating the brilliance of his fart-in plan when he explained the ins and outs of the tactic to *Playboy* magazine in 1972. The interesting thing is the fart-in protest idea survived the criticism of Vinson and lived on beyond the life of one of America's most famous radical agitators. His demonstration techniques were adopted for a great number of other causes. They also caught the attention of a young Barack Obama, who found Alinsky to be a source of interest in his own early career as a community organizer in Chicago.

Of course, Alinsky's record as a community organizer also has attracted the interest of critics on the ideological right in America. He has been demonized by extreme conservatives who have come to view him as the Anti-Christ who foments racial discord. It does not help that in his *Rules for Radicals*, Alinsky prefaces his work with an epigram celebrating Lucifer as "the first radical known to man who rebelled against the establishment." Not all radicals, including those fascinated by farts, would appreciate being lumped into the lineage of Lucifer. All of this begs the question: Are farts a divine gift to further the digestive processes of earthly creatures, or are they just another sordid weapon in the bottomless toolbox of Satan?

More Fart-In Musings

Barak Obama was not the only liberal and high-profile Democrat to find useful ideas in the rules established for radicals by activist Saul Alinsky. Hillary Clinton, who became the Democrats' nominee for U.S. president in the 2016 election, studied Alinsky's political movement techniques while she was a student at Wellesley College. She even wrote her thesis on his notions of radicalism in 1969; it was titled, "There Is Only the Fight: An Analysis of the Alinsky Model."[7]

Clinton interviewed Alinsky for her 1969 paper, and he offered her a place in his activist training school in Chicago. She opted instead for Yale Law School. Ironically, much later as a candidate for U.S. president in 2016, Clinton became a target for disgruntled Democrats who proposed using an Alinsky tactic against the former secretary of state and New York senator. Supporters of Clinton

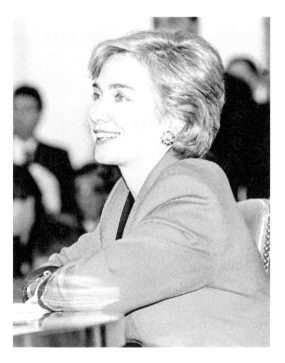

In the 2016 Democratic Primary, supporters of candidate Bernie Sanders organized a "fart-in" protest against the eventual nominee, Hillary Clinton. The Bernie Bros said their invisible flatulence demonstration would dramatize an unfair "illusion of democracy" in the race for the presidential nomination (Library of Congress).

rival Bernie Sanders decided to support a fart-in protest against Clinton at the Democratic National Convention in Philadelphia.

Just hours after Sanders conceded defeat in the 2016 presidential primary in July and endorsed his opponent Clinton, his hardcore supporters indicated that they would not go away quietly. Instead, the so-called "Sanderistas" said they would stage a noisy fart-in to protest Clinton's nomination at Philadelphia's Wells Fargo Center. The Poor People's Economic Human Rights Campaign vowed to collect a wide variety of donated canned and dried beans at its Philadelphia office. A plan was hatched to feed flatulence-inducing vegetables to willing Sanders supporters before they entered the convention hall.

The plan was attributed to longtime community organizer Cheri Honkala of the human rights campaign and she told the press it was designed to draw attention to the issue of income inequality and the plight of poor people in Philadelphia. The organization's actions started July 25 with a "March for Our Lives." Honkala said it was time to "demand an end to unemployment, hunger and homelessness; money for education; affordable, accessible housing; living wages; and an end to the prison industrial complex."[8]

Three days later the Beans for Hillary meal opened with an interdenominational prayer.

Honkala, a former vice presidential candidate for the Green Party, told the alternative media outlet *TruthDig* that "the Sanders delegates, their bellies full of beans, will be able to return to the Wells Fargo Center and greet the rhetorical flatulence of Hillary Clinton with the real thing."

Honkala explained that the fart-in is intended to demonstrate that "the [Democratic primary] process stinks." She stressed that farting is "non-violent" and the idea for the Philly fart-in arose organically from the "Sanderistas."

As with the original fart-in protest devised by community activist Alinsky in Rochester, New York, the concept was more effective at attracting media attention than in being effectively executed with any concrete results. The problem with fart-ins is that participants do not digest beans and vegetables at the same rate and the meals do not always produce the intended results. What's more, it's difficult to coordinate or synchronize the messages of fart-ins. Reporters in the national press were advised to keep an eye out—and a nose out—for queasy-looking Bernie-or-Bust diehards, but they should not hold their breath waiting for anything substantial to happen.

The 2016 presidential race ended in a contest between Democrat Hillary Clinton and Republican Donald Trump. After Trump lost the popular vote in America by almost three million votes, he still procured the presidency through the electoral college. Trump became the object of demonstrations, protests and occasional fart-ins by his frustrated opposition. Some of those fart-ins took place in Europe, where Trump was especially loathed. A protest in London included the famed Trump Baby Blimp and a giant farting Trump robot tweeting from a gold toilet.

The 16-foot robot was put in place in Trafalgar Square while the blimp was airborne over Westminster. The spectacle was meant to coincide with Trump's visit to London and his meetings with British officials. Demonstrators carried protest signs along with rolls of toilet paper featuring the president's image. The London *Independent* reported that the looming "Dump Trump" robot emitted farts and the American president's most notable quotes, including "I'm a very stable genius," "You are fake news," and "No collusion."[9]

Prior to the fart-ins aimed at Hillary Clinton and Donald Trump, the University of Texas at Austin witnessed a fart-in on the campus in 2015. The fart-in was actually a counter-demonstration against a gun rights group coming to campus that December to promote the idea that guns can make the campus safer. The pro-gun group brought cardboard guns and fake blood, and the sounds of gunshots played over bullhorns.

University of Texas alumnus Andrew Dobbs caught wind of the event. His response was to plan his own fart-in demonstration in response. Dobbs said he was tired of people trying to scare other people into thinking guns can make us safer. According to Dobbs, it was time for some good-hearted fart fun and a little humor as an antidote to the sounds of gun shots and carrying guns, whether fake or real.

Dobbs showed up on the UT campus with about 100 protesters, according to the *Houston Chronicle*. They shouted, "Texas farts!" and "We fart in your general direction." They marched through Austin with dildos, which are illegal on the university's campus. University of Texas professors have sued on several occasions to end laws passed by the state legislature allowing guns to be carried on campus but not unloaded dildos. In addition to wielding dildos the protesters carried devices that generated a variety of flatulence noises.

University officials breathed a sigh of relief that the farting protesters never crossed paths with pro-gun members of Come and Take It Texas and the DontComply.com group. A mock shooting by pro-gun groups was over by the time demonstrators arrived. A confrontation could have proven nasty, if not deadly. Past precedents reveal that such confrontations never clear the air of anything, whether the air is full of lead or flatulence. Though there was no feared confrontation, the anti-gun, fart-in group remained defiant.

"I choose to believe that fear is not the solution to the threat of our time. That laughing in the face of fear is a courageous act, and toting a gun around everywhere you go, maybe not so much," Dobbs said. "When you come to my community, to the university that I love, and you threaten the lives of my friends, what I have to say is: I'm going to fart in your face!"[10]

Alpha vs. Incel Farters

In addition to fart-ins and mass flatulence actions, there are the individual acts of flatulence rebellion. Two dramatically different kinds of men engage in flatulence demonstrations. One such man is the sexually active, physically healthy, alpha male. He has a superior appearance and displays a coveted physical prowess. The alpha male has it all. His brains and brawn are the bane and a source of bitterness for the angry incel man. The incel man has become characterized as an involuntary celibate with a boatload of resentments.

The alpha male farts loudly, confidently, and defiantly. He is telling the world through his manly fart to never doubt him,

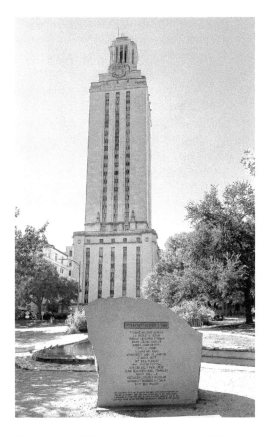

University of Texas at Austin, site of the 1966 campus tower shootings that took 18 lives, has been the location of many protests. A fart-in on campus in 2015 took aim at pro-gun groups, and a protest spokesperson declared: "When you come to my community, to the university that I love, and you threaten the lives of my friends, what I have to say is: I'm going to fart in your face!" (photograph by Leigh Muzslay Browne).

because he is exceptional and entitled. The alpha male will not tolerate either condescension or reprobation for his dramatic farting. He dealt it—and the world must smell it—because it is his right to anally announce his presence and to make his existence known. In other words, the alpha male is the rebel who says: "I am here and you better deal with it, because you have no other choice."

The incel man is not confident about anything, including his farts. He gives off puny fizzlers that give away his lack of physical stature and dearth of spirit. They are indicative of the incel's innate inferiority complex. Farts by incels are acts of nihilistic rebellion, carelessly released to send an incoherent message that, because the world does not give a hoot about them, they do not give a fig about the world. In fact, they insist the world has shortchanged them. Women worth having are not interested in them, and alpha males barely acknowledge that they exist.

The problem with the fizzler-farting incels is that they can be unstable and dangerous. Since 2000, a number of extremely violent and deadly incidents have been attributed to the incel movement and its common resentments. A "hero" of some incels is Elliot Rodger, who went on a shooting spree in Isla Vista, California, in 2014. Among the dead were sorority women at the University of California at Santa Barbara. Rodger confessed that he wanted to punish women for rejecting him and to also hurt sexually active men because he envied them. He emailed a lengthy manuscript explaining his feelings and the document was posted on the Internet and became widely known as the incel manifesto.[11]

Incel chat groups and their Internet presence can be extremely disturbing, because their comments are misogynistic, full of dark humor, and hostile toward women. They have been labeled as "male supremacists," because even though they seem full of insecurity, they believe that they are entitled to sex with women simply because they are men. They are not intentionally celibate, but they believe the unfairness of a superficial world has relegated them to that status. Rodger's manifesto contained a number of references to being rejected by women and being taunted and bullied by men who were successful with women.

Incels are acutely aware of what they see as their own obvious genetic shortcomings. They also are painfully aware of how outclassed they are by the alpha males. In the lexicon of the incel, names are given to all the human prototypes. For example, a Chad is a popular, attractive man who is sexually successful with women. A Stacy is beautiful, blonde, curvy and desirable. A Becky refers to women who are less desirable. A Cuck is very often an incel, who might have a chance with a Becky, but she would dump him in a minute to be with a Chad.

These named characters can be found on incel Internet sites and chat groups with some regularity. Many other names and terms used are offensive and dehumanizing. The term "femoid" or "foid" is an abbreviation for female humanoid or "female human organism." Monitors of incel sites have noticed that the term "foid" far exceeds the use of the name Stacy when referring to women. However, Chad is the primary term used when referring to the handsome, sexually active men who lead lives that are the envy of every Cuck, the frequently "cuckolded" incel.

In a post on the blog, *We Hunted the Mammoth*, writer David Futrelle analyzes an incel forum for an article titled, "Fart Discrimination: The Most Insidious Form of Anti-Incel Oppression." Futrelle is flummoxed by the lengths to which incels will go to find "new excuses to be angry at women." He finds it appalling that incels contend "women enjoy it when a handsome Chad farts in her presence, hating farts only when they come from ugly incels or other undesirable men."[12]

In an imaginary conversation on the incel site, Futrelle records how a Stacy woman and a Becky woman trash incel men together and then long for a Chad to come and rescue them from a creepy guy's gross farts. Becky tells Stacy, "This ugly guy's fart smells like the corpses of rotten children. I think he's a cannibal pedophile. I saw this crime show on TV where these hot detectives captured a creepy guy's fart in a bottle to test it for human remains, we should alert the authorities before he claims another victim, I can tell by his unattractive face that he's a psychopath who's out for blood and craves children."

In other words, if a man is virile and handsome, his farts are savored by hot women who enjoy the fine aroma. If a man is a weak and unlovable incel, his farting should be reported to authorities—the Law and Order Special Fart Unit. "The only people in the world who talk or think like this are incels and other weirdo manospherans," Futrelle observes.[13] Yes, this incel banter is weird and deranged. In fact, it is so sick that one wonders whether it is the kind of "red flag" material that would warrant an intervention by mental health experts.

Some feminists have little patience for any men farting in the presence of women. Period. Whether the blast emanates from a handsome Chad or a pathetic Cuck—the farting is most often just another sign of toxic masculinity meant to humiliate and intimidate women. Aggressive male farting may be a cry of protest from a desperate incel man or a demonstration of the ultimate manliness of a puffed-up Chad. In either case, women should not tolerate this kind of bodily behavior when it's aimed at them indiscriminately and without any consent.

Farting by a Chad or a Cuck, an alpha male or an incel, can be a deranged form of expression and downright pathological. On the other hand, farts as a form of protest by either right-wing or left-wing political activists would seem relatively harmless. Given the current ideological rifts and polarization in U.S. society today, a peaceful fart-in by either political persuasion should probably be encouraged. Power to the people! A chicken in every pot! Beans for everyone!

CHAPTER 14

Waxing Philosophically
About Farts

Most hard-working, meat-farting, flag-waving Americans don't care about what some philosopher has to say about flatulence. Their perception of philosophers is not flattering: impractical, pompous navel-gazers who contribute nothing to society. Americans view themselves as pragmatic and practical. In fact, they might benefit from reading philosophers who've helped shape the best ideas on pragmatism, practicality, and utilitarianism. Instead, Americans are more apt to read or listen to sneering diatribes that lampoon and make fun of philosophers.

Ancient philosophers, academic authorities, and philosophy professors are all targets of derision and grist for the mill of ridicule by the public. When it comes to flatulence and the great philosophers, jocular blogs and websites exist for mocking the fart logicians and theoreticians. On these sites, Descartes is credited with the declaration: "I fart, therefore I am." Machiavelli is credited with the statement: "Tell everyone you will not fart, then fart anyway." Shopenhauer is credited with the adage: "All farts pass through three stages: First, they are ridiculed. Second, they are violently opposed. Third, they are accepted as self-evident."[1]

The great existentialist philosophers come in for scorn as well. This is because existentialists do not offer certainty but instead abandon us to a meaningless and absurd universe. Naturally, true believers want revenge, and so Kierkegaard is mocked for reportedly observing: "The number of potential ways in which one could fart are limitless, so much so that one could not even comprehend the sheer volume of ways to fart. Regrets about your farting-related decision are inevitable. If you fart, you will regret it. If you do not fart, you will regret it. You are damned if you fart and damned if you don't fart. You will never know until the end of your life whether you should have farted or not but by then, you will have farted or not farted already. There is just no way to tell whether or not you should fart until it is too late to fart or not fart."[2]

Americans who appreciate a great thinker with his feet on the ground would probably prefer Michel de Montaigne, premier philosopher of the French Renaissance. Montaigne influenced America's founders and the new country's early scribes. He eschewed abstraction and established a direct style that was insightful, playful, humble, and full of common sense. Montaigne believed that humor was an effective means for getting ideas across and for making ideas acceptable and even pleasurable for readers. His humorous touch sometimes relied on personal anecdote and self-mockery, which made him a popular essayist.

Montaigne was a cultural relativist who took a reasoned, middle-of-the-road position on farting in his essays. His view might be summarized as "judge not, lest ye be judged."[3] He provided accounts of the various fart practitioners of his time, including an anecdote about a 16th century Frenchman of his acquaintance. Montaigne's Francophile friend, who flaunted his flatulence, liked to make long, continuous rumbles whenever he needed to part with his gas. Presented with this, Montaigne gave flatulence thoughtful consideration and concluded that everyone farts, therefore it's unfair to judge someone who has farted, whether in public or in private.

Montaigne's tolerant and sympathetic viewpoint has not always been shared by the great stinker thinkers who came before and after him. There are easily as many philosophical positions on the issue of farting as there are great philosophers. In fact, proponents of modern-day existentialist thought can maintain two contradictory positions at once on farting—or anything. The indecision of Soren Kierkegaard, an eminent 19th-century Danish theologian cited as a founder of existentialism, is a philosopher who clearly waffled on the question of farting. In contrast, Montaigne brought some sanity, sympathy, and understanding to the issue of farting.

Montaigne studied the issue of flatulence in earnest and concluded that we are all victims of disobedient body parts. He likened the stormy and churlish behavior of the buttocks to the inconsistent and unreliable behavior of the front male member. Apparently, erectile dysfunction was as persistent a problem for the French of his time as it is for the modern American male of a new century. Montaigne mused about men trying to use their minds to "will" the body to behave in a correct and satisfactory way. One recollection of Montaigne notes:

> To vindicate the omnipotence of our will, Saint Augustine alleges that he knew a man who commanded his behind to produce as many farts as he wanted, and his commentator (Juan) Vives goes him one better with an example of his own time, of farts arranged to suit the tone of verses pronounced to their accomplishment; but all this does not really argue any pure obedience in this organ; for is there any that is ordinarily more indiscreet or tumultuous? Besides, I

know one so turbulent and unruly, that for forty years it has kept its master farting with a constant and unremitting wind and compulsion, as is thus taking him to his death.[4]

Alas, the human body is going to have its way when it comes to farting, according to Montaigne. He notes that Saint Augustine and the erudite commentator Juan Vives have given reports of men who can control their intestinal gas for creative effect. But in the end, the intestines, sphincter, and anus constitute a sort of bodily organ that is disobedient at best and impudent in the extreme. There is simply no organ of the human body that is as "indiscreet and tumultuous." Montaigne invites us to face the music, especially after a high fiber diet of beans and other legumes.

Although many Americans lean toward ingesting humorous fart fare like that offered by the clever and occasionally wise-cracking Montaigne, others are more interested in gorging on serious fart discussion and engaging in altercations over flatulence. For every American who wants to enjoy a belly laugh from fart talk, there are at least three others who want gravitas. They want to argue, to debate, to become angry, and to take sides on flatulence. For the argumentative, there are distinguished sources available for such repartee in the fart pronouncements of the libertarians and communitarians, philosophers who predictably disagree with each other.

Libertarians vs. Communitarians

Libertarian philosophers hold individual liberty and autonomy to be primary. The individual is imbued with rights that include life, liberty, freedom of speech and association, freedom of worship, equality under the law, and the freedom to pursue one's own conception of happiness, which might very well include profligate flatulence. America's founders were heavily influenced by the concepts of libertarian philosophers. That is evident with the inclusion of the famous 14 words of the First Amendment, which is front and center in the U.S. Constitution.

The political philosophy of libertarianism derives from the French philosopher Francois-Marie Arouet Voltaire, the English philosophers John Locke, John Milton and John Stewart Mill, and the Scottish economist Adam Smith. These great minds influenced the American statesmen Thomas Jefferson and Benjamin Franklin. Jefferson and Franklin were persuaded to take a laissez-faire approach to the various utterances and articulations of their fellow men, which was consistent with the thought of the eminent libertarian philosophers who preceded them.

Voltaire's commitment to free expression also influenced America's founders, especially Franklin and Jefferson. Voltaire attained a solid standing among free expression stalwarts, if for no other reason than his dramatic decree that has withstood the test of time. Voltaire famously declared that he might very well disapprove of the nature and content of your pronouncements, but he would defend to the death your right to declare them vigorously and in public. Champions of flatulence have eagerly embraced Voltaire's declaration in regard to gas passing. However disagreeable the content of your backside utterances, the right for you to release them is beyond dispute.

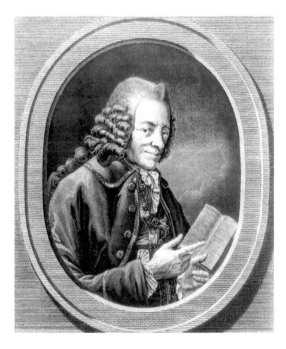

As a libertarian philosopher, Francois-Marie Arouet Voltaire might find your farting to be most disagreeable and reprehensible, but the intrepid Voltaire would certainly defend to his death your right to engage in all expressions of flatulence (Library of Congress).

John Milton's name often emerges when the subject of freedom of expression comes up. He is among the most-quoted advocates for a noisy liberty, even as other contemporaries counseled for peace and quiet. Milton's famous 1644 tract, known as *Areopagitica*, ignited a wave of demands for an end to suppression, both in Europe and America. Milton certainly did not hold back in his enthusiasm for the libertarian perspective: "And though all the winds of doctrine were let loose upon the earth, so truth be in the field, we do injuriously by licensing and prohibiting to misdoubt her strength."[5]

Given Milton's devotion to allowing the winds of ideas and doctrine to be let loose upon the earth, it is not a stretch to surmise that he would also approve of the mighty winds of flatulence to be unleashed upon the landscape. For those made uncomfortable by the breezes from the breach, Milton might suggest a clothespin or some other contrivance to pinch the nose shut. Of course, many of the offended would be more comfortable if somehow the door could be shut—even if only halfway—on noxious expression.

Milton was a believer in the "slippery slope" theory—that once you start restricting expression for the greater good, it's hard to know when or

where it will stop. Milton's concern with the slippery slope was shared by
many of the authors of the American Constitution. However, other American
commentators countered with a view toward the "social good." And
the social good may be something other than simply allowing everyone to
spout off anything, anywhere, at any time, from any orifice.[6]

Slippery slope or not, it's not too much of a hill to climb to conjecture
just how philosophers like Milton and Voltaire would come down
on the release of flatulence, particularly in view of their strong allegiance
to free expression. Likewise, it's not too much of a challenge to ascertain
where philosophers with reservations about free expression might come
down on the issue of unbridled flatulence. These thinkers are in the camp
that would counsel prudence, restraint, and self-discipline. These are
philosophic devotees to the primacy of the community and society—the
communitarians.

Premier among the notable intelligences of the past who would advocate
for caution, tact, and self-control on the issue of farting is the revered
sage K'ung-Fu-Tzu. Better known as Confucius, he lived in China from 551
to 479 BC. Confucius is the forerunner of the great communitarian philosophers
who, like Plato and Aristotle of Greece, championed collective
loyalty and subordination to the group. Communitarian thinkers of more
recent times might include Charles Fourier, Robert Owen, Alexis de Tocqueville,
and Karl Marx.

We know Confucius would frown on flatulence because of his emphasis
on the imperative of society over the autonomy of the individual. Social
order was extremely important for Confucius, and he felt the individual
must adapt and conform to its needs. According to Confucius, all virtue
disintegrates when individuals begin to act in an egocentric or self-indulgent
fashion. With the occurrence of this disintegration, "bravery
becomes foolhardiness or disobedience, frankness becomes rudeness or
vulgarity, and firmness becomes obstinance or eccentricity."[7]

Many complimentary descriptions can be applied to those who consider
the greater good of society and suppress their flatulence so as not
to offend others. Those favorable adjectives include unselfish, beneficent,
compassionate, considerate, and altruistic. Alternately, many uncomplimentary
descriptions can be applied to the gassy creatures who brandish
their flatulence and who show no concern about offending others. Those
unfavorable adjectives include selfish, uncaring, rude, and vulgar.

Confucius maintained that the glue holding society together is made
up of an amalgamation of cultural norms, approved customs, common
politeness, and basic manners. Without manners, life devolves into something
graceless, if not brutish. Insistence on everyday manners provides
a check on the undisciplined, anti-social behavior. Confucius would be

appalled at America's contemporary media with its incessant film creations rife with loud and obnoxious farting. Confucius would condemn the many pop culture products that capitalize on a vulgar fascination with the passing of gas.

Many centuries after the Chinese philosopher Confucius, British communitarian Alexis de Tocqueville came to America to study aspects of the fledgling libertarian democracy. America had broken with the traditions and manners of Tocqueville's Britain with a famous Declaration of Independence. America became a petri dish experiment of frontier spirit, crass materialism, rugged individualism, and diminished cultural norms. The English elites predicted that the new nation of "noble savages" would self-destruct in a cloud of gas after their departure from their British colony in the 1780s.

Tocqueville made astute travel commentaries on his visit to America in 1831. Tocqueville was impressed by America's egalitarianism, especially in contrast to the entrenched political power of European elites. However, he missed the civility and culture cultivated by the aristocracies of old Europe. Tocqueville felt the American citizenry's obsession with physical gratifications could lead to a loss of all self-constraints. He also questioned America's ability to produce genuine leaders. "Americans see themselves as farts from a rude ass and want to elect a fart from a rude ass," he declared.[8]

Tocqueville's 1835 remarks on America's "rude ass" echoed those of another British visitor to America named Charles Dickens. Both of them marveled at the seeming chaos, anarchy, dishonesty, and general lack of manners in the new land. Their writing makes it clear that they would raise their eyebrows, turn up their noses—and clothespin their nostrils tightly—at any free-wheeling displays of flatulence in a land of ruffians. Dickens held his nose when reading American newspaper accounts on the antics of the inhabitants. He wrote sarcastically that newsboys hawked newspapers in the streets yelling, "Here's the Sewer! Here's the Sewer!"[9]

Karl Marx was a contemporary of both Alexis de Tocqueville and Charles Dickens, an economics philosopher in Britain. Marx's critique of runaway capitalism in America echoed those of Tocqueville and the communitarians. However, Marx is more often characterized as a collectivist and communist than as a communitarian. Jokes about Marx's perspective on farts capitalize on his collectivism. For example, if Marx saw one man creating a lot of farts and another man producing very few farts, Marx would insist on redistributing the farts so that ownership became roughly equal.

Marx gained notoriety for his many associations with Europe's communitarian philosophers of the 19th century. Together the communitarians expressed contempt for mass production and what they viewed as the shoddiness of industrial capitalism. That contempt extended to the vulgar content of the advertising created to peddle inferior goods to the exploited masses. Another joke about Marx is that he viewed farts like he viewed religion, as an "opiate of the people," because an obsession with flatulence distracts the masses from organizing to improve their own lot in capitalist society.

A cursory glance at today's millions of dollars of fart games and fart toys available and sold on Internet sites certainly lends credence to the Marxian perspective. Marx might remark that a dearth of class consciousness and culture among the lower classes prevents their moving to the perfect gasless, classless society. Obsessed and amused with their gas and their many farting contrivances, the working classes are too distracted to mobilize for a proletarian revolution and a workers' paradise. Had Marx lived long enough to witness agitator Saul Alinsky's proletarian fart-ins for social justice causes, he may have found some hope in flatulence.

Existentialism: Angst and Farts

Moving on from Marx and other 19th-century philosophers, it is startling to learn how the views of many 20th-century existentialists are relevant to the ongoing milieu of flatulence. Among philosophers and writers counted as early existentialists are Soren Kierkegaard, Friedrich Nietzsche, Georg Wilhelm Hegel, Fyodor Dostoevsky, and William James. Existentialists of the 20th century, such as Hannah Arendt, Simone de Beauvoir, Franz Kafka, Karl Jaspers, Eugene Ionesco, Jean-Paul Sartre, Albert Camus, and Kurt Vonnegut, offer perspectives that are more pertinent to this discussion.

Modern existentialist writers Kafka, Ionesco, Sartre, Camus, and Vonnegut were especially popular among the counterculture college students of the 1960s and 1970s. During the latter decades of the 20th century, American college campuses were alive with students in thrall to existentialist ideas. The tumult of war protests, the civil rights movement, a music revolution, and the accessibility of hallucinogens were all factors prompting young people to reject the old order and to seek new answers to life's questions. There was a rejection of bourgeois cultural norms and manners.

College students of the time could be found on campus clutching such books as Kafka's *The Metamorphosis*, Ionesco's *Rhinoceros*, Sartre's *Nausea* and *No Exit*, Camus' *The Plague* and *The Myth of Sisyphus*, and Kurt Vonnegut's *Cat's Cradle* and *Slaughterhouse Five*. These books explored questions that all young people were asking: "What is the meaning of life? Why am I here? What is the purpose of existence? Why do I fart?" Writers and philosophers sought to answer these questions by examining such existential concepts as "the absurd," "facticity," "authenticity," and "angst and dread."

Revelations of the absurdity of life can be cathartic. The realization that life is absurd can be the beginning of a long journey in search of life's meaning. Avant-garde plays such as Ionesco's *Rhinoceros* can provide such a realization. The play is about the "rhinoceration" of good, ordinary people in the face of stress and anxiety. It mirrors the "Nazification" of average Europeans during the rise of the Third Reich. Kafka similarly probes the absurd with his story of a salesman who wakes up one morning to find he has been transformed into a giant cockroach. Kafka's *The Metamorphosis*, according to writer Vladimir Nabokov, is really about a creative man's struggles in a society filled with philistines intent on beating him down.[10]

Does it take the horror of seeing your friends transform into rhinoceroses to get a sense of the absurd? Maybe. However, seeing all your friends becoming unabashed gas passers could also be enough to trigger an existential epiphany. Is it necessary to wake up as a cockroach to discover life's absurdity? Maybe. But waking up with a hangover and a case of the green apple dirties, with gaseous side effects, can also be an existential wake-up call with cathartic and diarrhetic effect.

Existentialists spend their lives debating the meaning of life and describing the numerous absurdities of the human condition. Farts are clearly part of the human condition, with both men and women averaging a minimum of 12 to 15 flatus expulsions each and every day. And all of these fart expulsions serve to illustrate the absurdity of life. Humans have proclaimed themselves superior to Earth's creatures for centuries, yet many animals do not expel putrid, loathsome gases as humans do. Sloths do not fart. Octopuses do not fart. Birds do not fart. How absurd is it that belching, farting humans think of themselves as on a higher plane above all Earth's creatures?

Too many humans, especially today's variety of *Homo erectus*, no longer seem to even feel a sense of shame about accidental releases of gas in public spaces. Where once they were inclined to feel embarrassed, or even humiliated, they now find merriment in intentional gas passing. They pump up their chests as their posteriors deflate like punctured whoopee cushions. Humans revel in fart regalia, spending hundreds of dollars on fart sweatshirts, socks, hats, boxers, coffee mugs, iced tea glasses, and electronic fart simulators. How absurd is that?

From an existential standpoint, it's significant that humans come into this world with no capacity to control their sphincters. As babies, they fart, fume, and fill up their diapers. At some point, they mature and seem to take control of their lives. They struggle and strain for dignity, to achieve, and to try to make sense of it all. Like Albert Camus' character Sisyphus, they stumble, fall, and bruise as they push their heavy stone up the hill, only to lose control at the top and to watch it roll back down. And just as humans come into this life with no control of their sphincters, humans take their leave of this life once again lacking such control—filling their diapers and farting profusely. What's the point? How absurd is that?

Camus confronted absurdity with his literary account of a doctor dealing with a killer pandemic in Algeria. Sartre confronted absurdity with his literary account of a dejected history teacher who becomes physically nauseated by a meaningless life in his French town. Vonnegut confronted absurdity in his literary account of a troubled war veteran who becomes a successful optometrist and family man, only to be abducted by aliens called Trafalmadorians. All of these authors personally found meaning on their own mental slogs to the other side of despair.

However, Vonnegut never got over the absurdity of war and his own surreal experiences in World War II. Vonnegut survived a murderous three-day Allied carpet-bombing of Dresden that killed tens of thousands of German men, women, and children. Vonnegut was encapsulated three stories below the fiery carnage in the meat locker of a slaughterhouse. As an American POW, he lived through the carnage and was then ordered by his German captors to hunt for any sign of human life buried in the smoldering rubble. There was not much to rescue.

Vonnegut struggled mightily to make sense of his wartime experience and he suffered many fits of despair. He was appalled by the nuclear arms race and the development of a neutron bomb to kill people but to leave buildings and structures untouched. Vonnegut also was disturbed by the plight of his average fellow man, who often suffered the worst both in war time and in peace. He lamented that many American workers felt they were losing their purpose, because machines and computers were replacing them at their jobs and making them obsolete.

At the end of his life, Vonnegut counseled his fellow men to realize that their purpose was not about their jobs or their status but it was about being the eyes and ears and conscience of the universe. Vonnegut counseled his contemporaries to live by the Sermon on the Mount and to know that the meek shall inherit the earth. Above all, he counseled all human beings to not take themselves too seriously and to find happiness in each other. Today, a new generation of Americans wear shirts emblazoned with one of Kurt Vonnegut's most popular quotes: "I tell you we are here on earth to fart around and don't let anybody tell you different."[11]

Whirlwinds in His Bowels

American marvel Benjamin Franklin did not lead a life aligned with Kurt Vonnegut's proposition that "we are here on earth to fart around," although he had plenty to say on the subject of farts. Franklin was a mighty physical, political, scientific, and philosophical presence in the early years of the American experiment. He established himself in the colonies as an inventor, printer, editor, and essayist. The issues surrounding farting did not escape his earnest attention and sharp powers of observation.

As an inventor, Franklin gained much recognition for his work on stoves, fireplace inserts, reading glasses and bifocals and his outdoor experiments with electricity. Franklin was always looking for ways to improve our lives. In that respect, he could not leave the often sad situation with farting well enough alone. Franklin did not, however, desire to end the existence of the fart. He yearned for a fart of the future that would be pleasing to the senses. He accurately noted that in "permitting this Air to escape and mix with the Atmosphere, [it] is usually offensive to the Company, from the fetid Smell that accompanies it."[12]

Franklin observed that a dish of asparagus can make the urine smell bad. A dollop of turpentine can make the urine smell good. Using scientific method, he surmised that it therefore stands to reason that ingesting the right chemicals could alter the fragrance of a fart. Franklin's churning mind was always at work—whirling more than his own bowels. America's most unusual founding father was not farting around. Or was he? Maybe he was farting around!

In a letter to the Royal Academy of Brussels in Belgium, Franklin urged the distinguished body to take up his hypothesis. He requested that the Academy in Europe issue a call for scientific papers to take up the goal of discovering "some Drug wholesome & not disagreeable [*sic*], to be mix'd with our common Food, or Sauces, that shall render under natural Discharges of Wind from our Bodies, not only inoffensive, but agreable [*sic*] as Perfumes."[13]

Franklin's 1781 proposal to the Royal Academy is embodied in his essay "Fart Proudly." His fervent request was for scientists to create a concoction that would make farts smell swell. Franklin, who resided in Paris at the time, was greatly disappointed with what he viewed as the irrelevance of most research projects taken up by the scientific community. The philosopher of practicality did not actually send his proposal to the Royal Academy. He instead sent it to British scientist Joseph Priestley and radical pamphleteer Richard Price, heralded as the greatest thinker of Wales.[14] The American fart philosopher was interested in doing some shit-disturbing.

Franklin suggested an invention that transforms flatulence into an inviting fragrance would easily surpass all other scientific achievement and knowledge. He took a shot at René Descartes' formulation of a "Theory of Vortices." The popular theory held that outer space was filled with all kinds of matter whirling around the sun. Descartes believed that the universe was composed of a clockwork mechanism of vortical motion. It functioned perfectly and without intervention.

American iconoclast Franklin was not impressed by the work of French mathematician and philosopher Descartes. Franklin stated emphatically: "What Comfort can the Vortices of Descartes give a Man who has a Whirlwind in his Bowels!"[15] Franklin declared that when it comes to utilitarian value, all the revelations and discoveries of Aristotle, Newton, Descartes and others are "scarcely worth a FART-HING."[16] In retrospect, Franklin might have to concede that his own penchant for punning with the word "fart" was lacking.

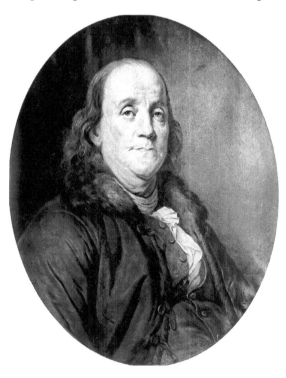

Founding father Benjamin Franklin has achieved immemorial status as the flatulence philosopher, thanks in part to his writing in "Fart Proudly." An inventor, Franklin sought a medical breakthrough to end the stench, but not the actual release, of colonial farts (Library of Congress).

Franklin's dream of a fragrant fart, thanks to human ingenuity, remains unrealized. Sadly, we do not yet possess the means to make farts smell as lovely as the freshly picked roses. We can take some comfort that drugs have been invented to reduce gas production. Research also has identified the offending foods which contain hydrogen sulfide such as beans, onions, cauliflower, broccoli, and dairy products. These items, plus red meat and raw eggs, disproportionately contribute to farts smelling badly. Franklin would not be so impressed by these findings.

Why did Franklin not want a medical invention that would end the reign of farts altogether? Why did he only want to get rid of the smell but not the vocalizations of the backside? Perhaps his orientation as a libertarian philosopher and a towering figure for free expression can explain this oddity. Franklin was not so hot on malodorous machinations, but he was a champion of free expression, whether originating from the heart and mind or the bowels and bunghole.

Franklin jested that it often did not make a difference where the noise and commotion comes from—because of the rough equivalency in intellectual weight of the content—from wherever the expression originates. He was devoted to free expression, regardless of its origin, regardless of who might take offense. Franklin said it was unreasonable to expect everyone to be pleased by the whirlwinds from an open mouth or the whirlwinds from an intestinal track exit.

Ben Franklin has recently been rediscovered and has found the spotlight in America. He is being recognized as America's own renaissance man. Celebrated filmmaker Ken Burns has produced *Ben Franklin*, an ode to the unique founding father. It's a four-hour documentary capturing the story of "the most famous American in the world" during the revolutionary era.[17] Also in production in 2022 was a cinematic series in which veteran actor Michael Douglas took up the challenge of playing the man known as the consummate politician, creative inventor, inveterate womanizer, and the grand old philosopher. Can his recognition as a champion of the almighty fart be far behind?

Franklin will always be the go-to man when it comes to American flatulence. He was far ahead of his time. In the wake of the Ken Burns' documentary on Franklin, commentators have suggested that Franklin seems like the founding father most likely to enjoy modern American life. "One can easily envision Franklin engaging in debates via blog, Twitter feed or TikTok," declared *Slate* writer Joseph Adelman.[18] With the limitations on verbiage imposed by Twitter, can anyone not imagine what Old Ben would tweet? For heaven's sake, just roar it out—and loudly: "Fart Proudly."

Postscript

For the Love of Farting

Throughout life's journey, flatulence makes its presence known. The continual escape of rectal gas is inescapable—it happens daily, nightly, during active waking hours and during the deepest of nocturnal slumbers. Obviously, a major portion of the human race insists on playing down the occurrence of farting. They dismiss it as simply an embarrassing inconvenience that should be ignored—it definitely should not be lionized or championed. However, there is another important segment of the human race that is fascinated—and at times obsessed—by the occurrence of flatulence. They're called "men."

For better or for worse, males seem to be the gender most often fixated and zeroed in on the release of gas. Men are acutely aware of their fascination and obsession from their own personal experiences. Every male can recollect extreme gas incidents in their life continuum. Some are more reticent to give voice to such memories; others revel in repeating and rehashing the most gruesome accounts. They will bring them up at every reunion and get-together of their male friends—brothers in a bond of male flatulence.

In this personal postscript, it seems appropriate to shed light on a just a few of my own encounters with memorable flatulence events. This final section has several functions. One of these functions simply involves freedom of information. Restraining gas can be painful and its release can be a source of relief to end discomfort. Likewise, suppressing or burying expulsion memories can be unhealthy, if not debilitating. It's therapeutic to liberate the mind of post-traumatic fart memories. It's important to share all manner of flatulence recollections.

A parallel function of this chapter is to provide insight into the rationale and inspiration for this definitive treatment of American flatulence. The flatulence in my own life's journey has inspired an attempt to answer a simple burning question: "Flatulence—what's it all about, Alfie?" Keep in mind that this autobiographical exercise does not use real names in most instances. The intent is to not invade anyone's privacy and to protect both the innocent and the guilty in assorted flatulence episodes.

My first encounter with the cultural relevance of flatulence—as well as the harsh taboos against flatulence expressions—came in second grade at Immaculate Conception School courtesy of Raymond Tarnowski. Little Raymond knew how to create astounding fart noises but not necessarily through his backside. He would spit saliva on his forearm, purse his lips on the slobbery wet spot, and blow off the loudest faux fart noises known to man. They would rattle the classroom windows at Immaculate Conception.

Tarnowski showed us youngsters how to summon hilarious faux farts, but most of us were afraid to laugh. Neither was the elderly nun laughing as Tarnowski disrupted her in the middle of her Catechism lesson on that paramount question: "Why did God make us?" Of course, the answer was "God made us to show His goodness and to share His everlasting happiness in heaven." There was not much happiness among the clerical authorities at Immaculate Conception after Raymond Tarnowski began ripping off big ones, albeit artificial and quite benign big ones.

Sister Mary Margaret called upon a higher power for help. She sought out the wrath of the parish priest, Father Beinert. The right reverend did nothing to de-escalate the crisis with Tarnowski. The Rev. Beinert knocked over Raymond's desk, dragged him by the earlobe up the classroom aisle, and disappeared with him out the classroom door. He was never seen or heard from again. We acolytes of the faith were startled—and left behind to wonder what happened to Tarnowski. Did he commit a venial sin? Did Tarnowski commit a mortal sin with his faux flatulence—a more serious offense against the laws of heaven? Was Raymond Tarnowski now exiled to purgatory or to the fires of hell itself? One thing was clarified for us: Farts are serious business. Keep them to yourself—real or otherwise.

Worry over the fate of Raymond Tarnowski, the trauma of the Catechism lesson interruption, and the sheer horror of second grade had worn off in just a few years. The great lesson of the second grade flatulence apocalypse was clearly unlearned. By fifth grade many of us Cub Scouts at the rank of Webelos were cutting our own rank, real cheese at Will—or George or Harry or whoever else was in the vicinity to be victimized. In fact, the dads of the boys of Immaculate Conception were to blame for our own memory loss and total loss of etiquette. Their hero was Babe Ruth, the Major League Baseball home run hitter, who perfected the "pull my finger" fart joke.

According to any popular culture dictionary definition, the "pull my finger" prank regarding flatulence occurs when a victim is asked to pull the finger of the joker, who simultaneously breaks wind so as to suggest a causal relationship between the two events. Cool, "in-the-know" fathers pulled this prank on their young sons as a rite of passage to adulthood in the 1950s and 1960s. However, David Hellweg's dad was not a cool, "in-the-know" father. So when he took his son and the rest of us Webelos on a memorable one-night camping trip, he was unprepared for what took place. There was a whole lot of finger-pulling going on past camping bedtime and into the wee hours of the morning.

It did not help that we Webelos had sat around the campfire, *Blazing Saddles*–style, eating pork and beans and barbecued hot dogs. David's dad tried to sleep on a cot in our very large tent, surrounded by us Webelos. The Webelos were filling sleeping bags with the detritus of newly-minted flatulence. To this day, there are recollections of David's dad retreating to his Ford Fairlane, swatting mosquitoes, trying to sleep through the night with his feet hanging out of the passenger-side window. He had brought us to the forest to hear the night calls of whippoorwills and the hoot owls. Instead, the evening was filled with the cry of barking spiders and ducks under foot, along with the giggles of young Webelos.

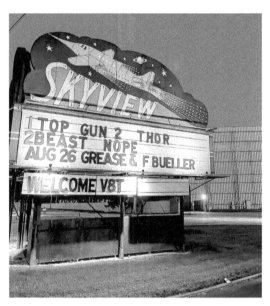

One way to get a free pass into the drive-in movie theaters of yesteryear was to ride in a car trunk past the ticket booth totally undetected. However, there was a price to pay if one of your companions in the car trunk was releasing tuna fish casserole gas (photograph by the author).

Not all dads drove Fairlanes or similar compact cars in our *Happy Days* era. Some dads motored around town in Lincoln Premieres and Chevy Impalas with eight-cylinder engines pulling giant car bodies sporting heavily-finned backside trunk spaces. The cars were subsequently driven by their entitled sons who graduated from the camp of the Webelos to the wonderland of teens with driver's licenses. Empowered teen boys got dad's car on weekends. They drove these cars with their cavernous trunks to partake in the thrill of drive-in theater scamming.

Years earlier, we boys had sat with mom and dad and sis in these giant cars to watch

Charlton Heston as Moses part the waters in *The Ten Commandments*. Now, we were going to see a barely-dressed Jane Fonda as *Barbarella* floating through space in her long black boots. But first we had to get past the drive-in ticket booth, with two guys in the front seat and three quiet guys in the car trunk. The trunk would be popped open inside the Skyview Theatre after two tickets were purchased. Then the sneak-a-show discounts would be applied equally for everybody.

Except that the guys in the trunk were not pleased with this arrangement. Especially after Steve Arbini released an air biscuit, then an ass flapper, and then a mum bomb as the carload of picture show poachers inched its way to the ticket booth in an endless line of cars. It was, indeed, painful, tortuous, excruciating. There was no escape from the fumes, and absolute silence had to be maintained. Arbini blamed his dog chimes and wet crank bugs on his mom's tuna fish casserole. His mother had no clue at dinner that, later in the evening, Steve Arbini's buddies would be gasping at breathing a gaseous mixture of her egg noodles, sordid chunks of Chicken of the Sea, rotten eggs and rancid mayonnaise flatulence—while locked in the trunk of a car.

By senior year in high school, Arbini's flatulence had taken a turn for the worse. Some incredible twisted pretzel farts replaced the tuna fish casserole farts of drive-in movie days. He had a job at Schulte's German Bakery Goods on Main Street, and every morning before school, he would roll thick strands of dough into enormous pretzels. The onion and honey mustard pretzels had an especially adverse impact on his malfunctioning innards. He ate tons of pretzels in the morning, which caused what Benjamin Franklin called a "stinking in the breeches" by the afternoon.

Steve Arbini's onion and honey mustard pretzel gas was bad enough in a high school classroom but even deadlier in the trunk of a Chevy Impala. That's right, we upstanding young men were once again riding in a cramped trunk. A group of us lived on Edgemont Hill in Illinois and we volunteered to tutor underprivileged children on English composition in nearby East St. Louis. It happened once a week after high school classes. This was in conjunction with one of President Lyndon B. Johnson's Great Society programs.

One difficulty was that parents did not want to volunteer their cars to transport us to what they felt was a dangerous locale, except for one owner of a Chevy Impala. He let his son borrow the car for the betterment of mankind and for the Great Society. To perform our community service, seven of us rode in his quickly deteriorating Impala on the way to East St. Louis. Four of us rode in the passenger compartment and three of us were made captive in the trunk. Two of us had to be in the closed compartment with the pretzel-rolling, onion-and-honey-mustard-tooting tutor, Steve Arbini.

Our work with underprivileged children served us well to obtain a community service credit. We put that on our applications to enter college, although it is questionable how much real knowledge we imparted on gerunds, infinitives, and participles to the children of East St. Louis. It's also doubtful that the college admission counselors had any real inkling as to what we endured to make the Great Society program happen. We were trapped in a gas-filled trunk with Steve Arbini to make it happen. The college admission counselors had no clue and never experienced even a brief whiff of an onion-and-honey-mustard-pretzel from a bowel howl from the tooting tutor, Steven H. Arbini.

Onto Higher Education

The college experience for male students of yesteryear, and today, often includes induction into a fraternity for a heavy dose of what has been termed the "Greek Life." In the past, fraternities have come in for serious criticism for elitism, favoritism, sexism, racism, homophobia, transphobia, xenophobia, alcohol abuse, academic dishonesty, hazing, and daily microaggressions against both pledges and active members. Fraternities can justifiably point out that they have taken steps to reform their *Animal House* image. They have attempted to become more accepting and multi-cultural and to be a more responsible part of the American collegiate scene.

Fraternities also like to point out that they can claim some responsibility for much of the leadership of the United States of America. Many fraternity members are in the corporate suites of the top Fortune 500 companies in the nation. Almost 40 percent of members of the U.S. Senate in recent years have been fraternity members. Many occupants of the White House have been fraternity members. Franklin Roosevelt, Gerald Ford, George W. Bush, George H.W. Bush, and Bill Clinton have all been initiated into fraternities.

Naturally, this writer wanted to enhance any potential to become the U.S. president or a corporate CEO and thus joined a fraternity pledge class to become a "Man of Tau" shortly after entering college. Fraternities initiate new members following a pledge period. The pledge period can involve secret rituals and memorization of Greek mysteries and sacred terminology. At the conclusion of an initiation, a Greek society's secret motto, secret identification signs, special handshakes, and passwords are revealed to the new members.

In addition to solemn rituals and arduous tests for membership, my own initiation to become a TKE involved much flatulence discussion and occasional farting microaggressions by active members of the fraternity. All members of the pledge class were forbidden to enter the fraternity house in a normal fashion but had to climb the front porch entrance stairs backward. We were not yet worthy to enter the house facing forward. We also had to recite an acknowledgment that even though we were "lower than whale farts, we were infinitely higher than any member of Phi Delta Theta."

After successfully completing an initiation and becoming something more than a whale fart, I was permitted to live in the college fraternity house. In the fraternity house, there was much flatulence discussion, regular farting microaggressions, and the infamous "Grosso Sandwich" ritual. This ritual involved two obese college football players who would strip down to their skivvies and engage in a long bout of sumo wrestling. The two wrestlers would grapple and tangle together in a mass of sweat, grunts, flatulence, and armpit odor. They would then hide in closets at either end of the second floor hallway of the fraternity house.

The second phase of the very gross sandwich ritual involved the two sumo wrestlers hiding in anticipation in the closets. They waited for an unsuspecting active or pledge to come walking down the hallway with his completed homework after an evening of "booking" in the library. At the right moment, the sumo wrestlers would suddenly emerge from the closets and begin primitive chanting as they begin to close in on a bookish, pre-med student like Laslo Farnsworth. They would clasp little Laslo between them in a "Grosso Sandwich," rubbing their sweat, body oils, and gaseous flatulence all over Laslo's pants, shirt, face and forehead.

Some of this unforgettable fraternity behavior, such as the "Grosso Sandwich," got in the way of my otherwise serious study as an English major. As an aside, it should be mentioned that my father questioned the efficacy and practicality of my being a "Man of Tau" as well as being an English major. Dad did this consistently at the end of every college semester. He might have felt otherwise if he had lived to see my current dissertation on flatulence.

The creation of this work would have been accelerated had my college professors been more aware of the common thread of flatulence in the fiction of great writers using the English language. The professors did mention, in passing, the classic fart scenes in the literature of Fielding and Chaucer. In retrospect, however, they might have served their English majors much better. They could have expounded on the critical literary tradition of flatulence among writers in both English and American literature. This English major caught wind of this flatulence tradition when writing a final college honors project, "The Picaresque Hero in the Works of Fielding, Twain, and Salinger." All three writers are wordsmith wonders in the flatulence literary tradition.

My educational enlightenment continued at the graduate school of journalism at the University of Missouri, where I was introduced to yet another flatulence writer and an author of the U.S. Constitution, Benjamin Franklin. Franklin has always been a hero and champion for journalists. A true universal man, Franklin advised journalists in his "An Apology for Printers" that writers should not have their feelings hurt if some readers find their work to be disagreeable or offensive. Wrote Franklin: "It is unreasonable in any one Man or Set of Men to expect to be pleas'd with everything that is printed, as to think that nobody ought to be pleas'd but themselves."

Franklin's observations on flatulence also are worthy of much study. He gave this journalist the spine and "internal fart-itude" to write without regret about a subject that should neither remain hidden nor couched in euphemism. Franklin advocated for expert methods to lessen the odorous effects of flatulence. He also described in minute detail the dietary requirements for avoiding, as well as for producing, a swarm of flatulence.

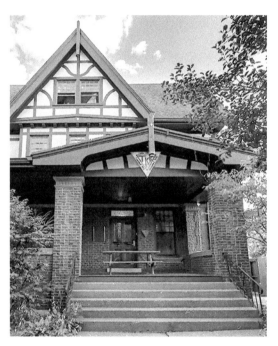

Wrote Franklin: "He that dines on stale Flesh, especially with much addition of Onions, shall be able to afford a Stink that no Company can tolerate; while he that has lived for some Time on Vegetables only, shall have that Breath so pure as to be insensible to the most delicate Noses, and if he can manage so as to avoid the Report, he may anywhere give Vent to his Griefs, unnoticed."

Freshman fraternity pledges were only permitted to climb the stairs backward to enter the Delta TKE Chapter House in Illinois in the 1960s. Pledges also had to recite a vow that, "even though I am lower in status than a whale fart, I know I will always be infinitely higher than any member of Phi Delta Theta" as they entered the House of Tau (photograph by Peter Bailley).

Doing Flatulence Journalism

A bit more than a decade after my first acquaintance with the honorable Benjamin Franklin, I followed in the great essayist's footsteps with my own journalistic observations on those who dine on stale flesh, particularly during the holidays. The article was titled "Holiday Diet & Stress Can Cause Gas," and it appeared in a great Midwest weekly newspaper in January 1992. The lead for this exposé was less flowery than Franklin's own prose but every bit as insightful.

The article began most auspiciously: "One of the undesirable after-effects of holiday stress and eating excess is the discomfort of bloating. That bloating is often a prelude to embarrassing gas or, more politely, flatulence." The front-page article included interviews with prominent St. Louis gastroenterologists Dr. John Eckrich and Dr. Charles J. Sigmund.

Gastroenterologist Eckrich noted that the problem of rectal gas can be addressed but cannot be entirely eliminated. He emphasized that the issue of unwanted gas emissions has been around for decades, centuries, maybe even eons. "We're talking about an age-old problem," said Eckrich. "If you go back to the ancient Greeks, in the Greek Senate, there were strict dietary rules aimed for the methane producers. They were not allowed to have beans or legumes during the senate session."

Sigmund observed that there are millions of chronic gas sufferers. For them, rectal gas is no laughing matter. On the other hand, Sigmund conceded there is a lighter side to the issue: "From time to time, I am kidded about my work at holiday cocktail parties. I'm called 'Dr. Sigmoid,' which refers to an area of the colon. I don't mind it."

Gastroenterologist Sigmund went back much further than the ancient Greeks to discuss the impact of rectal gas on terrestrial creatures. Sigmund noted: "There's a popular theory now that dinosaurs intoxicated themselves with their own methane. When you think about a million dinosaurs running around passing gas together, it's not an implausible theory."

The reception for the January 1992 article was mixed, with many readers expressing alarm to learn that the average person releases about a quart of rectal gas daily, or about 13 to 14 expulsions of various magnitude. One reader wrote about his amazement to learn that all normal, healthy people are passing a quart of the noxious gas per day, and he then remarked: "We're about a pint low—any suggestions?"

Among the other reader comments on the article about the heartbreak of flatulence:

- "One of the paper's better expulsions of journalism."
- "Hard-hitting investigative journalism at its best."

- "Bet you wore out your thesaurus on this one."
- "Exposes another attack on our liberties."

The Missouri state representative for the newspaper reading area, attorney Francis "Bud" Barnes, scribed a letter contending that there will always be a defense in court for objectionable gas passing in public venues. Wrote Barnes: "It is presumed by constitutional scholars that the defense of compulsion will always be available to any defendant (in fart offense cases). This defense basically says: 'I knew it was wrong, but I just had to do it.'"

Rep. Barnes presented this article writer with his own treasured volume, *Le Pétomane* by Jean Nohain and F. Caradec, a book that was a blockbuster among American readers. Also received was a lifetime supply of Beano from AkPharma, Inc., which instructed that Beano drops added to the first bite of an offending food will break down the powerful gas-producing sugars and prevent bloating, gas, and discomfort.

Not all the reactions to the article "Holiday Diet & Stress Can Cause Gas" were as laudatory or as charitable. Some readers demanded an apology to the community and that the editor be relieved of his position. They argued that the article was inappropriate and embarrassing for readers of a family newspaper, especially at the holidays. The attacks on the article and its author continued for several weeks. The diatribes may have precipitated my acid reflux which would demand serious treatment in a matter of years.

The doctors cited in the article, however, were most appreciative. They said the article was the first newspaper recognition of their work and their specialty. They noted other medical conditions that get extensive media treatment, while chronic flatulence is ignored because the subject makes people uncomfortable, if not upset. This all makes news editors want to keep flatulence in the closet. Readers want any discussion of the subject to be off-limits—confined to the doctor-patient relationship.

Some stories will haunt their writers for years, and that was surely the situation in my case with the holiday flatulence exposé. The unexpected and polarized reactions were stunning. From one quarter came lavish praise and gratitude. From the other quarter came ridicule and denunciation. Of course, these kinds of harsh responses only increased in my years of journalism that followed, as any edgy subject matter could set off agitated and highly opinionated readers. Controversy and consternation resulted in an agitation in my abdomen.

At some point, my acid reflux was aggravated to the extent that treatment was needed. Doctors were concerned that internal impacts could lead to esophageal cancer or other medical issues. I was prescribed both an upper GI endoscopy and a lower GI endoscopy. These both were performed on the same morning after I was sedated to reduce my discomfort and anxiety. The upper GI was intended to find narrowing strictures or blockages. The lower GI was basically a colonoscopy meant to check out the large intestine, colon, rectum, and anus for bleeding, ulcers, polyps, and suspected tumors.

After the endoscopies, I was wheeled into large room shaped like a wheel. The nurses' desk was at the axle. At the end of the spokes from that axle were recovery rooms each with a curtain for patient bed privacy. Like all the patients in the recovery room, who had endured the invasive colonoscopy, I was farting up a storm. Everybody was breaking wind in recovery. It was a flatulence rock concert with sounds ranging from heavy metal to glam to punk rock to Britpop. There were prostate poofs, hippo hiccups, steaming duffies, barking spiders, quake makers, fanny floaters, and more.

Naturally, my devoted spouse could not wait for me to regain consciousness and for the doctor to arrive to give a prognosis and then give us the green light to leave the symphony. I finally rustled to consciousness and began to reduce my own contribution to the concert in progress. For me, this symphony was a tribute to modern medicine and the attending physicians and nurses. Lives were being saved and improved here. In my anesthetic stupor, I began to fantasize having old Ben Franklin at my side as he enjoyed the melodies with me from a wide assortment of instruments. The hills were alive with the sound of music.

As I roused from my unconscious state, I realized that my "Benjamin Franklin" was actually the doctor, the specialist in gastrointestinal diseases, who worked his magic with his training in colonoscopy. The doctor offered a few observations on my chances for future bouts with colorectal cancer and esophageal cancer. I was mostly in the clear. He had removed a few benign intestinal polyps, but otherwise things were copacetic. There would only need to be a few dietary changes and modifications of sleeping habits. After the consultation, it was time to bid adieu to the melodious post-colonoscopy cacophony now made of honking horns—tubas, trombones, saxophones, clarinets, flutes, flugel horns and perhaps a few bagpipes.

As I was driven home, I was left with many of the same thoughts I had after my journalistic encounter of several years before with "Holiday Diet & Stress Can Cause Gas." I recalled the doctors who lamented that the media pay so little attention to their specialty. These are the unsung heroes of the cacophony of our honking horns. They are the essential plumbers of our vulnerable human anatomy. As a journalist, I resolved to do better by them. And I will do my best to urge my colleagues in the media to do so as well.

Self-Evident Flatulence Truths

When my associates, relatives, and friends learned that I was going to embark on this current flatulence writing adventure, some were dismayed, if not horrified. "It's good your mother is not alive to see this," one remarked. Others protested: "How could you devote four decades of your life to being a respected newspaper editor and accomplished journalism professor, and then cap it all off with an extended rant on farting?"

My rejoinder: I declare emphatically that a well-researched foray into flatulence is a valiant endeavor. If the topic was worthy of inclusion in the great literary legacy of Chaucer, Fielding, Shakespeare, Swift, Twain, and Salinger, then it is good enough for this dabbler in letters. If the topic had enough gravitas for a father of our country, Benjamin Franklin, then it is good enough for any humble scribe.

I do not shrink or cower at the criticism, but nothing causes me more annoying acid reflux regurgitations than to find I have devoted my energies to reading a lengthy book only to realize that I have learned nothing— that no useful lessons have been imparted. Readers who have indulged me thus far with their patience in reading such entries as "Fanning the Flames of Fart Conspiracies" and "Waxing Philosophically About Farts" deserve some concluding wise counsel and practical advice from the writer. So here, dearest readers, are some parting thoughts:

- Bring flatulence out of the closet or wherever else it lurks. Listen to it, analyze it, discuss it—maybe even enjoy it. Farting is important. Consider that kings and queens once found flatulence entertaining in their royal courts. If they could not get the real thing, they resorted to devices like whoopee cushions. Consider that chronic flatulence has affected the demeanor of generals and tyrants and thus changed the course of historic battles and wars.
- Popular culture has done much to normalize flatulence and to transform its fleeting winds into permanent subject matter for humor and delight. Film in particular has given us so many astonishing portrayals of flatulence emissions. Flatulence has launched the careers of our great stand-up comedians and there's more to come—both flatulence and comedy. Those hilarious movies have raked in billions of dollars, in part, by capitalizing on fart gags. It's been good for the American economy. Flatulence provides a portion of our Gross National Product.
- Respect and acknowledge the good work of physicians and other health professionals in the field of flatulence. America gives undue attention to cosmetic plastic surgeons but gives far less attention

to the doctors who keep the human plumbing and gas works functioning. Americans spend fortunes on surgery for breast augmentation, liposuction, tummy tucks, facelifts, nose reshaping, and eyelid surgery. Belly reductions and enlarged boobs have their place, but they are not necessarily essential for a rewarding life. Gastroenterologists merit much more attention for their good works. If flatulence is not brought under control, the expensive facelift and breast augmentation are all for naught in the quest to be attractive and desirable.

- Take a stand for free expression and against the censorship of flatulence expressions. Authoritarians always seek to put the lid on all farting because they do not find it flattering or edifying. It's embarrassing for their subjects to find out that not only does the king have no clothes, but the king also farts a lot. Older leaders have gas after every royal meal. The king is simply human. The populace needs to know that leaders and royalty put their pants on one leg at a time, often while farting. It's simply human.

- Avoid making farts an obsession or a fetish. This advice may appear to be hypocritical after releasing tens of thousands of words on the topic of flatulence. Regardless, this recommendation is serious. Constant chatter about farting is boorish and unpleasant. If you are constantly expelling gas, you need a gastroenterologist. If you are constantly farting, and talking about farting, you may need a psychologist and a clothespin. Flatulence fetishes are rare but not unheard of. Eproctophiles, who are usually male, reportedly spend inordinate amounts of time thinking about farting and having sexual fantasies about being farted upon. If you think you have this condition, go to a sex counselor who has a clothespin handy.

- Avoid all inclinations to weaponize flatulence in the continuing cultural, social, and political wars that plague us. It's a sad commentary on our times that farting became a heated controversy at the height of the recent pandemic. On the political front, conservatives attack liberals for permissiveness and for introducing children's fart books into schools. Conservatives speculate that this is a way to "groom" future eproctophiles. It's also part of a conspiracy to destroy good manners and societal norms. Liberals attack conservatives as sedentary old white men sitting in front of their Fox News while consuming cheese balls and brews—and cutting noxious beer farts. This profile may be accurate, but can we please just make flatulence a political debate-free zone?

- Turning to the gender war front, flatulence scholars and concerned professors engage in a lot of fruitless discussion on whether female farts smell worse than male farts. Additional intellectual query focuses on whether a male, who turns the wedding night bed into a ghastly Dutch oven, is transgressing with unwanted male domination. Is it an act of toxic masculinity? Has a woman, who actually relishes this farting, lost the most basic traits of the feminine mystique? Or is she actually a feminist? In any case, can we please make flatulence a gender war demilitarized zone?
- Never lose sight that flatulence is a completely natural phenomena that goes back eons to our evolutionary ancestors. Humans fart. What's more, bears do it, goats do it, baboons do it, monkeys do it, chimpanzees do it, hippos do it, and cows especially do it. Sloths don't do it. (What's wrong with those guys?) Sloths have a sedentary lifestyle in the trees, munching entirely on leaves. Their exceptionally slow-moving digestive system means they have no real need to fart. Sloths can justifiably blame everyone else in the forest for all the gas passing.
- Sloths may be the only mammal not to fart, but the rest of us mammals are picking up the slack. Global human population is growing at an alarming rate. The population has exploded from a mere one billion in 1800 to about eight billion in 2020 to a projected 11.2 billion by 2100. We billions of humans are farting more than a trillion of gallons of rectal gas into the atmosphere on an annual basis. We cannot say "excuse me" nearly enough times to make amends. We cannot begin to be good stewards of the earth if we fart wantonly and excessively.

A first step in addressing our atmospheric flatulence problem is awareness. An awareness of our excessive gas production will not only help us address the collective global rectal gas crisis, but this awareness will also make us more cognizant of our own humanity. We do have our inevitable indiscretions. When we recognize our humanness, our vulnerability, our flatulence and our mortality, we will do better as creatures with responsibilities to each other and our planet.

Humans come into this world farting into a diaper, and if they are fortunate to grow old enough, they take their leave of this world farting into a diaper. Mark Twain recognized this more than a century ago. Gas is just a fact of life—and death. Yet, how many friends and relatives have we witnessed in their final hours trying to deny their flatus? In their futile attempts to deny it they are mortified. They try to hold it back to the end. It's pitiful, humiliating, and unnecessary. We must comfort them and tell them it's okay. It's time to sing to them a final anthem of acceptance, perhaps the poignant and moving song from Disney's *Frozen*: "Let It Go."

The holy man applies ashes to our foreheads on Ash Wednesday and speaks these words: "Remember that thou are dust, and to dust you shall return." The practice is meant to impart knowledge of our vulnerability, our helplessness in the face of eternal forces, our basic collective humanness. The practice should include a subtext: "We come into this world farting into a diaper—and if we are fortunate to grow old enough—we leave this world farting into a diaper. And that is okay. Let it go. Let it go."

Chapter Notes

Chapter 1

1. Joshua Rhett Miller, "'Panera Karen' Claims Masks Won't Stop COVID-19 Since Pants Don't Contain Farts," *New York Post*, July 22, 2020, https://nypost.com/2020/07/22/panera-karen-masks-dont-stop-covid-19-since-pants-dont-contain-farts/.

2. Joshua Rhett Miller, "'Panera Karen' Claims Masks Won't Stop COVID-19 Since Pants Don't Contain Farts," *New York Post*, July 22, 2020, https://nypost.com/2020/07/22/panera-karen-masks-dont-stop-covid-19-since-pants-dont-contain-farts/.

3. David A. Lieb and James Salter, "Missouri Governor, Opponent of Mandatory Masks, Has COVID-19," *Associated Press*, September 23, 2020, https://apnews.com/article/virus-outbreak-us-news-mo-state-wire-michael-brown-ap-top-news-ec3963a041c3061abba62493aa0bb2be.

4. Joshua Rhett Miller, "'Panera Karen' Claims Masks Won't Stop COVID-19 Since Pants Don't Contain Farts," *New York Post*, July 22, 2020, https://nypost.com/2020/07/22/panera-karen-masks-dont-stop-covid-19-since-pants-dont-contain-farts/.

5. Joshua Rhett Miller, "'Panera Karen' Claims Masks Won't Stop COVID-19 Since Pants Don't Contain Farts," *New York Post*, July 22, 2020, https://nypost.com/2020/07/22/panera-karen-masks-dont-stop-covid-19-since-pants-dont-contain-farts/.

6. Jen Christensen, "New Studies Agree That Animals Sold at Wuhan Market Are Most Likely What Started COVID-19 Pandemic," *CNN*, July 27, 2022, https://www.cnn.com/2022/07/26/health/wuhan-market-covid-19/index.html.

7. Joshua Rhett Miller, "'Panera Karen' Claims Masks Won't Stop COVID-19 Since Pants Don't Contain Farts," *New York Post*, July 22, 2020, https://nypost.com/2020/07/22/panera-karen-masks-dont-stop-covid-19-since-pants-dont-contain-farts/.

8. Bruce Lee, "Can Farts Transmit COVID-19 Coronavirus? Here Is What Is Being Said," *Forbes*, April 27, 2020, https://www.forbes.com/sites/brucelee/2020/04/27/can-farts-transmit-covid-19-coronavirus-here-is-what-is-being-said/?sh=50137e82310f.

9. Ananya Mandal, "Lifting the Lid on Coronavirus Flatulence," *News Medical Life Sciences*, April 22, 2020, https://www.news-medical.net/news/20200422/Lifting-the-lid-on-coronavirus-flatulence.aspx.

10. Alexandra Sternlicht, "Why You Should Flush with the Lid Down: Experts Warn of Fecal-Oral Transmission of COVID-19," *Forbes*, April 2, 2020, https://www.forbes.com/sites/alexandrasternlicht/2020/04/02/why-you-should-flush-with-the-lid-down-virologist-warns-of-fecal-oral-transmission-of-covid19/?utm_campaign=forbes&utm_source=facebook&utm_medium=social&utm_term=Valerie%2F&sh=2a2aeec26eb8.

11. "Hot Air?" *BMJ* 323(7327), December 22, 2001, https://www.ncbi.nlm.nih.gov/pmc/articles/PMC1121900/.

12. Rhett Allain, "If Masks Work, Why Can I Smell Farts?" *Geek Physics*, May 28, 2020, https://medium.com/geek-physics/if-masks-work-why-can-i-smell-farts-c0b8e10323c6.

13. Caydiid Ali, "Coronavirus 'could be spreading across the globe through farts' Claim Doctors," *The Daily Star*, April 12, 2020, https://www.allbanaadir.org/?p=149490.

14. Ron Dicker, "Stephen Colbert Has a Gas with Doctor's Warning on Farts Spreading Coronavirus," *HuffPost*, April 22, 2020, https://www.huffpost.com/entry/stephen-colbert-farts-coronavirus_n_5ea01b0dc5b6b2e5b83a913a.

15. Bruce Lee, "Can Farts Transmit COVID-19 Coronavirus? Here Is What Is Being Said," *Forbes*, April 27, 2020, https://www.forbes.com/sites/brucelee/2020/04/27/can-farts-transmit-covid-19-coronavirus-here-is-what-is-being-said/?sh=50137e82310f.

Chapter 2

1. Dave Bonta, "Slow Life," Via Negativa, February 21, 2004, https://www.vianegativa.us/2004/02/slow-life/.

2. Gregory Ryskin, "Methane-driven Oceanic Eruptions and Mass Extinctions," *GeoScienceWorld*, September 1, 2003, https://pubs.geoscienceworld.org/gsa/geology/article-abstract/31/9/741/29324/Methane-driven-oceanic-eruptions-and-mass.

3. Gregory Ryskin, "Methane-driven Oceanic Eruptions and Mass Extinctions," *GeoScienceWorld*, September 1, 2003, https://pubs.geoscienceworld.org/gsa/geology/article-abstract/31/9/741/29324/Methane-driven-oceanic-eruptions-and-mass.

4. Jim Dawson, *Blame It on the Dog* (Berkeley: Ten Speed Press, 2006), 92–93.

5. Jim Dawson, *Who Cut the Cheese?* (Berkeley: Ten Speed Press, 1999), 27.

6. Nick Caruso and Dani Rabaiotti, *Does It Fart? The Definitive Guide to Animal Flatulence* (New York: Hachette Books, 2018).

7. Deborah Bunting, "Ministry That Built Life-Size Noah's Ark Will Rebuild Tower of Babel to Glorify God, Combat Racism," *CBN News*, November 12, 2021, https://www1.cbn.com/cbnnews/entertainment/2021/november/ministry-that-built-life-size-noahs-ark-will-rebuild-tower-of-babel-to-glorify-god-combat-racism.

8. Malcolm Gladwell, *David and Goliath: Underdogs, Misfits and the Art of Battling Giants* (New York: Little Brown and Company, 2015).

9. "Clarence Darrow's Examination of William Jennings Bryan at the 1925 Scopes Trial," *Beliefnet*, https://www.beliefnet.com/news/science-religion/1999/12/clarence-darrows-examination-of-william-jennings-bryan-at-the-1925-scopes-trial.aspx.

10. Candida Moss, "How a Fart Killed 10,000 People," *The Daily Beast*, July 23, 2019, https://www.thedailybeast.com/how-a-fart-killed-10000-people.

11. Candida Moss, "How a Fart Killed 10,000 People," *The Daily Beast*, July 23, 2019, https://www.thedailybeast.com/how-a-fart-killed-10000-people.

12. Kahlid Elhassan, "The Fart That Killed 10,000 People, and Other Weird Moments from History," *History Collection*, July 18, 2020, https://historycollection.com/the-fart-that-killed-10000-people-and-other-weird-moments-from-history/2/.

13. Peter Preskar, "Adolf Hitler Farted Like a Horse," *medium.com*, May 2, 2021, https://medium.com/short-history/adolf-hitler-farting-b7e27477971b.

14. Miles Klee, "Bill O'Reilly and Jimmy Kimmel Chat About Hitler's Farts," *Daily Dot*, February 10, 2015, https://www.dailydot.com/upstream/bill-oreilly-kimmel-hitler-farts/.

15. Richard Brennan, "Ugly Americans, Farting Their Way to Alienation," *eats shoots 'n leaves blog*, August 6, 2010, https://richardbrenneman.wordpress.com/2010/08/06/ugly-americans-farting-their-way-to-alienation/.

16. Ron Dicker, "Jimmy Fallon Rips Savage Lines About Rudy Giuliani Farting During Hearing," *HuffPost*, December 4, 2020, https://www.huffpost.com/entry/jimmy-fallon-rudy-giuliani-fart_n_5fca0b47c5b63a153450eff4.

17. Dwight Garner, "Stop the Steal, Giuliani's Flatulence, a Reichstag Moment," *The Irish Times*, July 22, 2021, https://www.irishtimes.com/culture/books/stop-the-steal-giuliani-s-flatulence-a-reichstag-moment-trump-s-apocalyptic-final-year-1.4625864.

18. George Dvorsky, "We've Grossly Underestimated How Much Cow Farts

Are Contributing to Global Warming," *Gizmodo*, September 29, 2017, https://gizmodo.com/we-ve-grossly-under estimated-how-much-cow-farts-are-con-1818993089.

19. Staff Report, "Doctors Petition White House to Cut U.S. Meat Production to Tackle Climate Crisis," *Good Medicine*, Spring 2021, 10.

20. Antonia Noori Farzan, "The Latest Right-Wing Attack on Democrats: 'They want to take away your hamburgers,'" *Washington Post*, March 1, 2019, https://www.washingtonpost.com /nation/2019/03/01/latest-right-wing-attack-democrats-they-want-take-away-your-hamburgers/.

Chapter 3

1. Carl Japiske, ed., *Fart Proudly: Writings of Benjamin Franklin You Never Read in School* (Columbus, OH: Enthea Press, 1990) 13–17.

2. Carl Japiske, ed., *Fart Proudly: Writings of Benjamin Franklin You Never Read in School* (Columbus, OH: Enthea Press, 1990) 13–17.

3. "Watch Out, Pokemon. After Conquering Japan, the Yo-kai Are Here to Invade Europe," *Stuff.TV*, April 20, 2016, https://www.stuff.tv/review/yo-kai-watch-review/.

4. Baud's Advice Column, "Help, I'm Dating the Barking Spider," *Metafilter.com*, July 29, 2007, https://ask.metafilter.com/68077/Im-dating-the-barking-spider.

5. Angry Topaz, "Was That a Barking Spider?" *Roller Mountain Girls: Denver*, 2020, https://rockymountainrollergirls.com/member-of-the-month-barking-spider/.

6. Martin S. Weinberg and Colin J. Williams, "Fecal Matters: Habitus, Embodiments, and Deviance," *Semantic Scholar*, August 2005, https://www.semanticscholar.org/paper/Fecal-Matters%3A-Habitus%2C-Embodiments%2C-and-Deviance-Weinberg-Williams/3be7a980af0ba2beb7c722e681af3c24650da9d1.

7. George Dvorsky, "We've Grossly Underestimated How Much Cow Farts Are Contributing to Global Warming," *Gizmodo*, September 29, 2017, https://gizmodo.com/we-ve-grossly-under estimated-how-much-cow-farts-are-con-1818993089.

Chapter 4

1. Elizabeth Bromstein, "Hold Those Fart Jokes," *NOW*, July 3, 2017, 1–2, https://nowtoronto.com/hold-those-fart-jokes.

2. F. Azpiroz, *Intestinal Gas* (Philadelphia: Elsevier, Inc., 2021) 224–231; see also M. Feldman, et. al., eds. *Sleisenger & Fordtran's Gastrointestinal and Liver Disease*. 11th Edition.

3. E. Thursby and N. Juge, "Introduction to the Human Gut Microbiota," *Biochemical Journal* vol. 474, no. 11 (May 2017): 1823–1836. https://pubmed.ncbi.nlm.nih.gov/28512250/.

4. F.L. Suarez and M.D. Levitt, "An Understanding of Excessive Intestinal Gas," *Current Gastroenterology Reports* vol. 2, no. 5 (October 2000): 413–419. https://pubmed.ncbi.nlm.nih.gov/10998670/.

5. D.A. Drossman, Z. Li, E. Andruzzi, R.D. Temple, N.J. Talley, W.G. Thompson, W.E. Whitehead, J. Janssens, P. Funch-Jensen, E. Corazziari, J.E. Richter, and G.G. Koch, "U.S. Householder Survey of Functional Gastrointestinal Disorders," *Digestive Diseases and Sciences* vol. 38, no. 9 (September 1993): 1269–1580. https://pubmed.ncbi.nlm.nih.gov/8359066/.

6. D.K. Chitkara, A.J. Bredenoord, M.J. Rucher, and N.J. Talley, "Aerophagia in Adults: A Comparison with Functional Dyspepsia," *Alimentary Pharmacology and Therapeutics* vol. 22, no. 9 (November 2005): 855–858. https://pubmed.ncbi.nlm.nih.gov/16225495/.

7. A.C. Ford and N.J. Talley, "Irritable Bowel Syndrome," M. Feldman, et. al., eds., *Sleisenger & Fordtran's Gastrointestinal and Liver Disease*. (Philadelphia: Elsevier, Inc., 2021), 2008–2020.

8. M. Pimentel, R.J. Saad, M.D. Long, and S.C. Rao, "ACG Clinical Guideline: Small Intestinal Bacterial Overgrowth," *The American Journal of Gastroenterology* vol. 115, no. 2 (February 2020): 165–178. https://journals.lww.com/ajg/fulltext/2020/02000/acg_clinical_guideline__small_intestinal_bacterial.9.aspx.

9. G.A. Weiss and T. Hennet, "Mechanisms and Consequences of Intestinal

Dysbiosis," *Cellular and Molecular Life Sciences* vol. 74, no. 16 (August 2017): 2959–2977. https://pubmed.ncbi.nlm.nih.gov/28352996/.

10. B. Giovanni, M. Grover, P. Bercik, M. Corsetti, U.C. Ghoshal, L. Ohman, and M.R. Rajilic-Stojanovic, "Rome Foundation Working Team Report on Post-infection Irritable Bowel Syndrome," *Gastroenterology* vol. 156, no. 1 (January 2019): 56–58. https://pubmed.ncbi.nlm.nih.gov/30009817/.

11. J.M. Shapiro and J.K. Deutsch, "Complementary and Alternative Medicine Therapies for Irritable Bowel Syndrome," *Gastroenterology Clinics of North America* vol. 50, no. 3 (September 2021): 671–688. https://pubmed.ncbi.nlm.nih.gov/34304794/.

Chapter 5

1. "What Does Breaking Wind Mean?" *Writing Explained*, Accessed August 15, 2022, https://writingexplained.org/idiom-dictionary/breaking-wind.

2. Andrew Sullivan, "A History of Farting," *The Atlantic*, July 18, 2007, https://www.theatlantic.com/daily-dish/archive/2007/07/a-history-of-farting/226692/.

3. Luke Holm, "An Analysis of 'The Miller's Tale' in Geoffrey Chaucer's *The Canterbury Tales*," *Owlcation*, July 8, 2022, https://owlcation.com/humanities/An-Analysis-of-The-Millers-Tale-in-Geoffrey-Chaucers-The-Canterbury-Tales.

4. William Shakespeare, *The Comedy of Errors* (New York: CreateSpace Independent Publishing, 2016).

5. Henry Fielding, *The History of Tom Jones—a Foundling, Penguin Classic* (New York: Penguin Classics, 2005).

6. Jonathan Swift, "The Benefit of Farting Explain'd," *Booktryst*, May 17, 2012, http://www.booktryst.com/2012/05/jonathan-swift-on-women-who-fart-or.html.

7. Jonathan Swift, "The Benefit of Farting Explain'd," *Booktryst*, May 17, 2012, http://www.booktryst.com/2012/05/jonathan-swift-on-women-who-fart-or.html.

8. Nadja Spiegelman, "James Joyce's Love Letters to His 'Dirty Little Fuckbird,'"
The Paris Review, February 2, 2018, https://www.theparisreview.org/blog/2018/02/02/james-joyces-love-letters-dirty-little-fuckbird/.

9. Alexia Walker, "English Literature vs. American Literature," *The Adroit Journal*, May 1, 2019, https://theadroitjournal.org/2019/05/01/english-literature-vs-american-literature/.

10. Carl Japiske, ed., *Fart Proudly: Writings of Benjamin Franklin You Never Read in School* (Columbus, OH: Enthea Press, 1990), 13–17.

11. Carl Japiske, ed., *Fart Proudly: Writings of Benjamin Franklin You Never Read in School* (Columbus, OH: Enthea Press, 1990), 13–17.

12. Mark Twain, *1601: Conversation, as It Was by the Fireside in the Time of the Tudors* (Belpre, OH: Blennerhasset Press, 1914).

13. Mark Twain, *1601: Conversation, as It Was by the Fireside in the Time of the Tudors* (Belpre, OH: Blennerhasset Press, 1914).

14. Gary Scharhorst, *The Life of Mark Twain 1891–1910* (Columbia: University of Missouri Press, 2022), 227–228.

15. Earnest Hemingway, *Earnest Hemingway 88 Poems*, edited by Nicholas Gerogiannis (New York: Abe Press, 1979).

16. Jim Dawson, *Who Cut the Cheese?* (Berkeley: Ten Speed Press, 1999), 42–43.

17. J.D. Salinger, *The Catcher in the Rye* (New York: Bantam Books, 1978), Chapter 3.

18. J.D. Salinger, *The Catcher in the Rye* (New York: Bantam Books, 1978), Chapter 3.

Chapter 6

1. Dawn McMillan, *My Butt Is So Noisy* (Mineola, NY: Dover Publications, 2021).

2. Sylvia Branzei, *Grossology: The Science of Really Gross Things* (New York: Price Stern Sloan, 2002).

3. Lisa Ferland, "Why We Need More Kids' Books About Farts," *Lisa Ferland Consulting* blog, June 20, 2019, https://lisaferland.com/books-about-farts/.

4. Jane Bexley, *Freddie the Farting Snow Man* (Independently Published, 2020).

5. Jane Bexley, *Dad and Me Setting Farts Free* (Independently Published, 2021).

6. Humor Heals Us, *Fritz the Farting Reindeer* (Middletown, DE: Humor Heals Us Publishing, 2020).

7. Jane Bexley, *Princesses Don't Fart (They Fluff)* (Independently Published, 2021).

8. Tootin' Tom, *My Dad Loves to Toot* (Tootin' Tom's Books, 2021).

9. Leanne Italie, "How to Get Boys to Read? Try a Book on Farts," *Associated Press*, July 21, 2010.

Chapter 7

1. Marshall McLuhan and Quentin Fiore, *The Medium Is the Message* (New York: Bantam Books, 1967) 1–10.

2. Nancy Mead, "Sermon: 'Whatever happened to class,'" *Alamosa News*, May 25, 2018, https://alamosanews.com/article/sermon-whatever-happened-to-class.

3. Angelique Chrisafis, "Scotland Yard Recoils from a Foul Wind," *The Guardian*, June 6, 2001, https://www.theguardian.com/uk/2001/jun/07/angeliquechrisafis.

4. "Man in Court After Deliberately Farting at Police and Asking 'How do you like that?,'" *The Scotsman*, September 20, 2019, https://www.scotsman.com/news/crime/man-court-after-deliberately-farting-police-and-asking-how-do-you-1407196.

5. "Fugitive Caught After Blowing His Cover with Fart," *BBC News*, May 7, 2020, https://www.bbc.com/news/uk-england-nottinghamshire-52577485.

6. Sam Blitz, "Breaking Wind, Breaks Cover! Suspect hiding in bushes is caught by police after letting off a fart," *Daily Mail*, May 8, 2020, https://www.dailymail.co.uk/news/article-8301289/Breaking-cover-Man-hiding-bushes-police-gave-away-letting-FART.html.

7. David Moye, "Suspect's Loud Fart Helps Police Sniff Out His Hiding Place," *HuffPost*, July 10, 2019, https://www.huffpost.com/entry/farting-suspect-arrested-liberty-missouri_n_5d2602a6e4b07e698c441405.

8. Daniel Chaitlin, "'Hate to cause a stink': FCC Chairman Declines to Investigate Alleged Swalwell Flatulence," *Washington Examiner*, November 19, 2019, https://www.washingtonexaminer.com/news/hate-to-cause-a-stink-fcc-chairman-
declines-call-to-investigate-alleged-swalwell-flatulence.

9. Daniel Chaitlin, "'Hate to cause a stink': FCC Chairman Declines to Investigate Alleged Swalwell Flatulence," *Washington Examiner*, November 19, 2019, https://www.washingtonexaminer.com/news/hate-to-cause-a-stink-fcc-chairman-declines-call-to-investigate-alleged-swalwell-flatulence.

10. Harvey Silverglate, "Obscenity v. Indecency in the Eyes of the Supreme Court," *Boston Phoenix*, May 13, 2005, https://bostonphoenix.com/boston/news_features/other_stories/documents/04689746.asp.

11. Damien Cave, "Media Fights for Free Speech," *Rolling Stone*, May 11, 2004, https://www.rollingstone.com/music/music-news/media-fights-for-free-speech-236224/.

12. Matthew Lasar, "Clear Channel to FCC: Wash XM-Sirius' Mouth Out with Soap," *ArsTechnica*, March 25, 2008, https://arstechnica.com/uncategorized/2008/03/clear-channel-to-fcc-wash-xm-sirius-mouth-out-with-soap/.

13. Matthew Lasar, "Clear Channel to FCC: Wash XM-Sirius' Mouth Out with Soap," *ArsTechnica*, March 25, 2008, https://arstechnica.com/uncategorized/2008/03/clear-channel-to-fcc-wash-xm-sirius-mouth-out-with-soap/.

14. Matthew Lasar, "Clear Channel to FCC: Wash XM-Sirius' Mouth Out with Soap," *ArsTechnica*, March 25, 2008, https://arstechnica.com/uncategorized/2008/03/clear-channel-to-fcc-wash-xm-sirius-mouth-out-with-soap/.

Chapter 8

1. Jean Nohain and F. Caradec, *LePetomaine* (Los Angeles: Sherbourne Press, 1967), 7–8.

2. Jean Nohain and F. Caradec, *LePetomaine* (Los Angeles: Sherbourne Press, 1967), back cover.

3. Jean Nohain and F. Caradec, *LePetomaine* (Los Angeles: Sherbourne Press, 1967), 8–15.

4. Taylor McAdams, "'Blazing Saddles' Producers Hid These Facts from the Public," BrainSharper, September 16, 2019,

https://www.brain-sharper.com/entertainment/blazing-saddles-tb/34/.

5. Nancy Churnin, "Something New Is in the Air for the Karamazovs," *Los Angeles Times*, June 12, 1992, https://www.latimes.com/archives/la-xpm-1992-06-12-ca-186-story.html.

6. Kathleen Krull and Paul Brewer, *Fartiste* (New York: Simon & Schuster, 2008).

7. A.A. Crist, "InterAct Theatre Presents the World Premiere of SETTLEMENST," *Broadway World*, March 4, 2022, https://www.broadwayworld.com/philadelphia/article/InterAct-Theatre-Presents-The-World-Premiere-Of-SETTLEMENTS-20220304.

8. Jay Reiner, "Rousing 'Can-Can' Puts the Kick Back in Vintage Show," *Hollywood Reporter* (Reuters), July 6, 2007.

9. Carly Stern, "Thousand Year History of Flatulists," *Daily Mail*, March 8, 2018, https://www.dailymail.co.uk/femail/article-5474797/The-history-flatulists-comedic-fart-performers.html.

10. Jim Dawson, *Who Cut the Cheese?* (Berkeley: Ten Speed Press, 1999), 134.

11. Jim Dawson, *Who Cut the Cheese?* (Berkeley: Ten Speed Press, 1999), 132–33.

12. Brian Lowry, "'George Carlin's American Dream' Finds the Right Words to Capture the Comedy Icon," *CNN*, May 20, 2022, https://www.wral.com/george-carlins-american-dream-finds-the-right-words-to-capture-the-comedy-icon/20291431/.

13. Matt Wilstein, "What Jon Stewart Learned About Fart Jokes from George Carlin," *Daily Beast*, May 19, 2022, https://finance.yahoo.com/news/jon-stewart-learned-comedy-george-013733822.html.

14. Jason Diamond, "Judd Apatow on Documenting the Legacy (and Fart Jokes) of George Carlin," *Vulture*, May 2022, https://www.vulture.com/2022/05/judd-apatow-george-carlin-documentary-interview.html.

15. Jason Diamond, "Judd Apatow on Documenting the Legacy (and Fart Jokes) of George Carlin," *Vulture*, May 2022, https://www.vulture.com/2022/05/judd-apatow-george-carlin-documentary-interview.html.

16. Storm Gifford, "Eddie Murphy Wins First Emmy for 2019 'Saturday Night Live' Return," *New York Daily News*, September 19, 2020, https://www.nydailynews.com/snyde/ny-eddie-murphy-wins-first-emmy-20200920-tgnx3yo6b5filex3qggenc2une-story.html.

17. Joel Keller, "Eugene Miriman," *AV Club*, March 28, 2012, https://www.avclub.com/eugene-mirman-1798230562.

18. Deborah Solomon, "Making Nice," *The New York Times*, August 20, 2006, https://www.nytimes.com/2006/08/20/magazine/20wwln_q4.html.

19. Joseph Lesmi, "How Many Times Has 'The View' Star Whoopi Goldberg Hosted the Oscars?" *Showbiz Cheatsheet*, August 27, 2020, https://www.cheatsheet.com/entertainment/how-many-times-has-the-view-star-whoopi-goldberg-hosted-the-oscars.html/.

20. Dan Glaister, "Goldberg Dropped from Diet Ads over Bush Joke," *The Guardian*, July 16, 2004, https://www.theguardian.com/world/2004/jul/16/uselections2004.film.

21. Olivia Cole, "Whoopi Goldberg Reminds Us That Women Fart Too—and That's OK," *Bigmouth* blog, January 27, 2015, https://oliviaacole.wordpress.com/2015/01/27/whoopi-goldberg-reminds-us-that-women-fart-too-and-thats-ok./.

22. Kate Brierley, "Meet 'The Soup's' Newest Host Jade Catta-Preta," *Distractify*, https://www.distractify.com/p/jade-catta-preta-the-soup.

23. Thom Jennings, "Comedian Nikki Glaser Not All She Appears," *Niagara Gazette*, October 15, 2014, https://www.niagara-gazette.com/news/night_and_day/comedian-nikki-glaser-not-all-she-appears/article_3cbe0924-18ae-5f5f-835e-67012d99ec67.amp.html.

24. Jason Zinoman, "The Strategic Mind of Ali Wong," *New York Times*, May 3, 2018, https://www.nytimes.com/2018/05/03/arts/television/ali-wong-netflix-hard-knock-wife.html.

25. Nayomi Reghay, "Meet the Trans Comedian Making Fart Jokes an Act of Resistance," *Rolling Stone*, October 13, 2017, https://www.rollingstone.com/culture/culture-features/patti-harrison-meet-the-trans-comedian-making-fart-jokes-an-act-of-resistance-196357.

Chapter 9

1. Ethen Reese, "The Darling Meaning of 'Hakuna Matata' from 'The Lion King'

for Parents," *American Songwriter*, July 2022, https://americansongwriter.com/the-darling-meaning-of-hakuna-matata-from-the-lion-king-for-parents/.

2. Robert Alan Crick, *The Big Screen Comedies of Mel Brooks* (Jefferson, NC: McFarland, 2002), 64–66.

3. Owen Gleiberman, "The Nutty Professor," *Entertainment*, June 28, 1996, https://ew.com/article/1996/06/28/nutty-professor-2/.

4. Roger Ebert, "Women Can Get Drunk and Be Crude Too," *Roger Ebert*, May 11, 2011, https://www.rogerebert.com/reviews/bridesmaids-2011.

5. Lee Nathan, "Parody Without Plot in 'Scary Movie 4,'" *New York Times*, April 14, 2006, https://www.nytimes.com/2006/04/14/movies/parody-without-plot-in-scary-movie-4.html.

6. Jim Sullivan, "Sex, Comedy Are Main Dishes Served with 'American Pie,'" *The Boston Globe,* September 4, 2014, http://ae.zip2.com/boston/scripts/staticpage.dll?only=y&spage=AE%2Fmovies%2Fmovies_details.htm&id=20376&ck=&ccity=Massachusetts&cstate=MA&adrVer=889718808&ver=e2.7.

7. Daryl H. Miller, "Alan Smithee Makes a Name in Hollywood," *Los Angeles Times,* March 5, 2002, https://www.latimes.com/archives/la-xpm-2002-mar-05-et-miller5-story.html.

8. "Carrie Fisher Helped Write 'Last Action Hero' and Six Other Things You Didn't Know About the Cult Classic," *yahoo*, June 18, 2018, https://www.yahoo.com/entertainment/carrie-fisher-helped-write-last-120000208.html.

9. "How Old Was Lloyd Bridges in the Movie 'Hot Shots! Part Deux'?" *inthatmovie.com*, accessed April 21, 2023, https://inthatmovie.com/2177-9255/lloyd-bridges/hot-shots-part-deux.

10. Lloyd Paseman, "Light Movie Funny, but Tasteless," *Eugene Register-Guard*, August 7, 1980, https://news.google.com/newspapers?id=XvhVAAAAIBAJ&sjid=5EDAAAAIBAJ&pg=6752%2C1975045.

11. Gene Siskel, "Siskel's Flick Picks," *Chicago Tribune*, March 25, 1988, https://www.chicagotribune.com/news/ct-xpm-1988-03-25-8803030550-story.html.

12. AP Review, "Carrey's 'Liar, Liar' Has Record Opening," *Observer-Reporter*, March 25, 1997, https://www.metacritic.com/movie/liar-liar.

13. Neil Gaiman and Kim Newman, *Ghastly Beyond Belief* (New York: Random House Group, 1985).

14. Peter Debruge, "Sundance Film Review: 'Swiss Army Man,'" *Variety*, January 22, 2016, https://variety.com/2016/film/reviews/swiss-army-man-film-review-1201685807/.

15. Ramin Setoodeh, "Sundance: Daniel Radcliffe's Farting Corpse Movie Prompts Walk-Outs," *Variety*, January 22, 2016, https://variety.com/2016/film/news/daniel-radcliffe-farting-corpse-swiss-army-man-1201686756/.

16. "Laura Esquivel Biography," *biography.com*, 2006, http://www.biography.com/search/article.do?id=185854.

17. Ethen Reese, "The Darling Meaning of 'Hakuna Matata' from 'The Lion King' for Parents," *American Songwriter*, July 2022, https://americansongwriter.com/the-darling-meaning-of-hakuna-matata-from-the-lion-king-for-parents/.

Chapter 10

1. Penny Chavers, "Whoopee Cushions and Prank Phone Calls: The Oldest Tricks in the Book," *Curious Historian*, July 31, 2019, https://curioushistorian.com/whoopee-cushions-and-prank-phone-calls-the-oldest-tricks-in-the-book.

2. Penny Chavers, "Whoopee Cushions and Prank Phone Calls: The Oldest Tricks in the Book," *Curious Historian*, July 31, 2019, https://curioushistorian.com/whoopee-cushions-and-prank-phone-calls-the-oldest-tricks-in-the-book.

3. Leo Braudy, Scott Higgins, Stephen Groening and Thomas Delapa, "Smell-O-Vision, Astro-color and Other Film Industry Inventions That Proved to Be Flops," *Smithsonian Magazine*, February 28, 2018, https://www.smithsonianmag.com/innovation/smell-o-vision-astrocolor-other-film-industry-inventions-that-proved-to-be-flops-180968295/.

4. National Park Service, "The Story of the Teddy Bear," *nps.gov/learn/history*, July 15, 2021, https://www.nps.gov/thrb/learn/historyculture/storyofteddybear.html.

5. Daniel Braff, "Why We Pass More

Gas as We Age," *AARP Magazine*, June 24, 2020. https://www.aarp.org/disrupt-aging/stories/info-2020-passing-gas.html.

Chapter 11

1. Earl J. Cyler, "Farting, Fellowship, Forgiveness," *Man-Making Blog*, February 23, 2013, http://journeytomanhood.blogspot.com/2013/02/farting-fellowship-and-forgiveness.html.

2. Earl J. Cyler, "Farting, Fellowship, Forgiveness," *Man-Making Blog*, February 23, 2013, http://journeytomanhood.blogspot.com/2013/02/farting-fellowship-and-forgiveness.html.

3. Chris Moss, "A Fine Bromance: The 12 Rules of Male Friendship," *The Telegraph,* January 13, 2017, https://www.telegraph.co.uk/men/relationships/a-fine-bromance-the-12-rules-of-male-friendship/.

4. Chris Moss, "A Fine Bromance: The 12 Rules of Male Friendship," *The Telegraph,* January 13, 2017, https://www.telegraph.co.uk/men/relationships/a-fine-bromance-the-12-rules-of-male-friendship/.

5. Michael Messner, *Politics of Masculinities: Men in Movements* (Thousand Oaks, CA: Sage, 1997), 11–13.

6. Michael Messner, *Politics of Masculinities: Men in Movements* (Thousand Oaks, CA: Sage, 1997), 16–19, 93–94.

7. Don Corrigan, "Promise Keepers: Men of Integrity," *Webster-Kirkwood Times* (St. Louis), October 27, 1995.

8. Michael Messner, *Politics of Masculinities: Men in Movements* (Thousand Oaks, CA: Sage, 1997), 64–80.

9. Warren Farrell, *The Myth of Male Power* (New York: Berkeley Books, 1993), 21–41.

10. Michael Messner, *Politics of Masculinities: Men in Movements* (Thousand Oaks, CA: Sage, 1997), 36–48.

11. Michael Messner, *Politics of Masculinities: Men in Movements* (Thousand Oaks, CA: Sage, 1997), 49–55.

12. Michael Messner, *Politics of Masculinities: Men in Movements* (Thousand Oaks, CA: Sage, 1997), 80–96.

13. Albert Riehle, "On Farting," *A Beast, an Angel, and a Madman* blog, September 16, 2007, http://albertriehle.blogspot.com/.

14. Albert Riehle, "On Farting," *A Beast, an Angel, and a Madman* blog, September 16, 2007, http://albertriehle.blogspot.com/.

15. Albert Riehle, "On Farting," *A Beast, an Angel, and a Madman* blog, September 16, 2007, http://albertriehle.blogspot.com/.

16. Richard Brennan, "Ugly Americans, Farting Their Way to Alienation," *eats shoots 'n leaves* blog, August 6, 2010, https://richardbrenneman.wordpress.com/2010/08/06/ugly-americans-farting-their-way-to-alienation/.

17. Gina Cavallaro, "For Marines in Afghanistan: Be Careful Where You Fart," *BattleRattle* blog, August 6, 2010, http://battlerattle.marinecorpstimes.com/2011/08/23/for-marines-in-afghanistan-be-careful-where-you-fart/.

Chapter 12

1. "Turns Out, Women's Farts Smell Worse Than Men's," *Men's Health*, May 1, 2021, https://www.menshealth.com.au/turns-out-women-s-farts-smell-worse-than-men-s/.

2. Ross Pomeroy, "Women's Farts Smell Worse, and Five More Facts You Need to Know About Flatulence," *RealClearScience* blog, October 2, 2014, https://www.realclearscience.com/blog/2014/10/6_facts_you_need_to_know_about_farts.html.

3. Bethany Brookshire, "Friday Weird Science: The Social Psychology of Flatulence," *Bethanybrookshire.com* blog, March 23, 2013, https://bethanybrookshire.com/friday-weird-science-the-social-psychology-of-flatulence/.

4. Glosswitch, "Why Farting Is a Feminist Issue," *New Statesman*, December 9, 2014, https://www.newstatesman.com/politics/2014/12/why-bodily-functions-are-feminist-issue.

5. Glosswitch, "Why Farting Is a Feminist Issue," *New Statesman*, December 9, 2014, https://www.newstatesman.com/politics/2014/12/why-bodily-functions-are-feminist-issue.

6. Bruce Y. Lee, "90 Day Fiancé Star Sells Her Farts in Jars Then Suffers Health Scare," Forbes, January 8, 2022, https://www.forbes.com/sites/brucelee/2022/01/08/90-day-fianc-star-sells-farts-in-jars-then-suffers-health-scare/?sh=b40929536fc3.

7. Bruce Y. Lee, "90 Day Fiancé Star Sells Her Farts in Jars Then Suffers Health Scare," *Forbes,* January 8, 2022, https://www.forbes.com/sites/brucelee/2022/01/08/90-day-fianc-star-sells-farts-in-jars-then-suffers-health-scare/?sh=b40929536fc3.

8. Peter Furz, *Tailwinds: The Language of Fizzles, Farts and Toots* (London: Michael O'Mara Books, 1998), 52.

9. Ross Scarano and Greg Topscher, "25 Laughable Sex Scenes from Famous Male Novelists," *Complex.com* blog, February 27, 2013, https://www.complex.com/pop-culture/2013/02/25-laughable-sex-scenes-from-famous-male-novelists/.

10. Tracy Moore, "If You Love Someone, Let Her Fart," *Mel Magazine*, April 7, 2017, https://medium.com/mel-magazine/if-you-love-someone-let-her-fart-616483145e52.

Chapter 13

1. Atoosa Moinzadeh, "Texas Protesters Hold 'Mass Farting' to Counter Pro-Gun Group's Fake Mass Shooting," *Vice*, December 12, 2015, https://www.vice.com/en/article/3kw5jb/texas-protesters-hold-mass-farting-to-counter-pro-gun-groups-fake-mass-shooting.

2. Liz Spikol, "Jewish Activist Alinsky Inspires Unconventional Protest Set for Convention's Final Afternoon," *Jewish Exponent*, July 20, 2016, https://www.jewishexponent.com/2016/07/20/jewish-activist-alinsky-inspires-unconventional-protest-set-for-conventions-final-afternoon/.

3. Eric Norden, "Saul Alinsky: Playboy Interview (March 1972)," *Scraps from the Loft* blog, May 1, 2018, https://scrapsfromtheloft.com/comedy/saul-alinsky-playboy-interview-1972/.

4. Eric Norden, "Saul Alinsky: Playboy Interview (March 1972)," *Scraps from the Loft* blog, May 1, 2018, https://scrapsfromtheloft.com/comedy/saul-alinsky-playboy-interview-1972/.

5. Irmin Vinson, "'So the last shall be first...' Alinsky's Farting Negroes," *Counter-Currents*, September 6, 2016, https://counter-currents.com/2016/09/alinskys-farting-negroes/.

6. Irmin Vinson, "'So the last shall be first...' Alinsky's Farting Negroes," *Counter-Currents*, September 6, 2016, https://counter-currents.com/2016/09/alinskys-farting-negroes/.

7. Liz Spikol, "Jewish Activist Alinsky Inspires Unconventional Protest Set for Convention's Final Afternoon," *Jewish Exponent*, July 20, 2016, https://www.jewishexponent.com/2016/07/20/jewish-activist-alinsky-inspires-unconventional-protest-set-for-conventions-final-afternoon/.

8. Liz Spikol, "Jewish Activist Alinsky Inspires Unconventional Protest Set for Convention's Final Afternoon," *Jewish Exponent*, July 20, 2016, https://www.jewishexponent.com/2016/07/20/jewish-activist-alinsky-inspires-unconventional-protest-set-for-conventions-final-afternoon/.

9. Alessio Perrone, "Trump Protests: Giant Model of President Sitting on a Golden Toilet While Tweeting Appears in Central London," *The Independent*, June 4, 2019, https://www.independent.co.uk/news/uk/home-news/trump-protests-toilet-robot-tweeting-trafalgar-square-london-state-visit-a8943061.html.

10. Atoosa Moinzadeh, "Texas Protesters Hold 'Mass Farting' to Counter Pro-Gun Group's Fake Mass Shooting," *Vice*, December 12, 2015, https://www.vice.com/en/article/3kw5jb/texas-protesters-hold-mass-farting-to-counter-pro-gun-groups-fake-mass-shooting.

11. Antonia Molloy, "California Killings: Elliot Rodger's parents knew of massacre on radio as they raced to stop their son," *Independent*, May 27, 2014, https://www.independent.co.uk/news/world/americas/california-killings-elliot-rodger-s-parents-heard-about-massacre-on-radio-as-they-raced-to-stop-their-son-9435197.html.

12. David Futrelle, "Fart Discrimination: The Most Insidious Form of Anti–incel Oppression?" We Hunted the Mammoth blog, November 15, 2018. https://www.wehuntedthemammoth.com/2018/11/15/fart-discrimination-the-most-insidious-form-of-anti-incel-oppression/.

13. David Futrelle, "Fart Discrimination: The Most Insidious Form of Anti–incel Oppression?" *We Hunted the Mammoth* blog, November 15, 2018. https://www.wehuntedthemammoth.com/

2018/11/15/fart-discrimination-the-most-insidious-form-of-anti-incel-oppression/.

Chapter 14

1. Tom Foolery, "Philosophers on Farting," *Bookshelf Battle*, June 23, 2017, https://bookshelfbattle.com/2017/06/23/philosophers-on-farting/.

2. Tom Foolery, "Philosophers on Farting," *Bookshelf Battle*, June 23, 2017, https://bookshelfbattle.com/2017/06/23/philosophers-on-farting/.

3. John C. Merrill, *Legacy of Wisdom* (Ames: Iowa State University Press, 1994), 37–40.

4. Michel de Montaigne, "Of the Powers of the Imagination," in *The Complete Works: Essays, Travel Journal, Letters.* Translated by Donald M. Frame. Everyman Library 259 (New York: Alfred A. Knopf, 2003), 87–88.

5. Calder M. Pickett, *Voices of the Past: Key Documents in the History of American Journalism* (New York: John Wiley & Sons, 1977), 8–11.

6. John C. Merrill, *Legacy of Wisdom* (Ames: Iowa State University Press, 1994), 41–44.

7. John C. Merrill, *Legacy of Wisdom* (Ames: Iowa State University Press, 1994), 3–9.

8. John C. Merrill, *Legacy of Wisdom* (Ames: Iowa State University Press, 1994), 79–83.

9. Calder M. Pickett, *Voices of the Past: Key Documents in the History of American Journalism* (New York: John Wiley & Sons, 1977), 83–84.

10. Mauro Nervi, "Lecture on 'The Metamorphosis' by Vladimir Nabokov" *The Kafka Project*, August 10, 2022.

11. Nicholas Lezard, "Farewell to the Master of Farting Around," *The Guardian*, April 12, 2007, https://www.theguardian.com/books/booksblog/2007/apr/12/farewelltoamasteroffartin.

12. Carl Japiske, ed., *Fart Proudly: Writings of Benjamin Franklin You Never Read in School* (Columbus, OH: Enthea Press, 1990), 13–17.

13. Carl Japiske, ed., *Fart Proudly: Writings of Benjamin Franklin You Never Read in School* (Columbus, OH: Enthea Press, 1990), 13–17.

14. Carl Japiske, ed., *Fart Proudly: Writings of Benjamin Franklin You Never Read in School* (Columbus, OH: Enthea Press, 1990), 13–17.

15. Carl Japiske, ed., *Fart Proudly: Writings of Benjamin Franklin You Never Read in School* (Columbus, OH: Enthea Press, 1990), 13–17.

16. Carl Japiske, ed., *Fart Proudly: Writings of Benjamin Franklin You Never Read in School* (Columbus, OH: Enthea Press, 1990), 13–17.

17. Joseph Adelman, "It's Finally Ben Franklin's Time in the Sun," *Slate*, April 4, 2022, https://slate.com/news-and-politics/2022/04/ben-franklin-ken-burns-review-michael-meyer-philanthropy.html.

18. Joseph Adelman, "It's Finally Ben Franklin's Time in the Sun," *Slate*, April 4, 2022, https://slate.com/news-and-politics/2022/04/ben-franklin-ken-burns-review-michael-meyer-philanthropy.html.

Bibliography

Adelman, Joseph. "It's Finally Ben Franklin's Time in the Sun." *Slate,* April 4, 2022. https://slate.com/news-and-politics/2022/04/ben-franklin-ken-burns-review-michael-meyer-philanthropy.html.

Ali, Caydiid. "Coronavirus 'could be spreading across the globe through farts' Claim Doctors." *The Daily Star,* April 12, 2020. https://www.allbanaadir.org/?p=149490.

Allain, Rhett. "If Masks Work, Why Can I Smell Farts." *Geek Physics,* May 28, 2020. https://medium.com/geek-physics/if-masks-work-why-can-i-smell-farts-c0b8e10323c6.

Bart, Benjamin. *The History of Farting.* London: Michael O'Mara Books Limited, 1993.

Blitz, Sam. "Breaking Wind, Breaks Cover! Suspect hiding in bushes is caught by police after letting off a fart." *Daily Mail,* May 8, 2020. https://www.dailymail.co.uk/news/article-8301289/Breaking-cover-Man-hiding-bushes-police-gave-away-letting-FART.html.

Braff, Daniel. "Why We Pass More Gas as We Age." *AARP Magazine,* June 24, 2020. https://www.aarp.org/disrupt-aging/stories/info-2020/passing-gas.html.

Branzei, Sylvia. *Grossology: The Science of Really Gross Things.* New York: Price Stern Sloan, 2002.

Bromcie, Alec. *The Complete Book of Farting.* London: Michael O'Mara Books Limited, 1999.

Bromstein, Elizabeth. "Hold Those Fart Jokes." *NOW,* July 3, 2017. https://now toronto.com/hold-those-fart-jokes.

Caruso, Nick, and Dani Rabaiotti. *Does It Fart? The Definitive Guide to Animal Flatulence.* New York: Hachette Books, 2018.

Cavallaro, Gina. "For Marines in Afghanistan: Be Careful Where You Fart." *Battlerattle,* August 6, 2010. http://battlerattle.marinecorpstimes.com/2011/08/23/for-marines-in-afghanistan-be-careful-where-you-fart/.

Cave, Damien. "Media Fights for Free Speech." *Rolling Stone,* May 11, 2004. https://www.rollingstone.com/music/music-news/media-fights-for-free-speech-236224/.

Chaitlin, Daniel. "'Hate to cause a stink': FCC Chairman Declines to Investigate Alleged Swalwell Flatulence." *Washington Examiner,* November 19, 2019. https://www.washingtonexaminer.com/news/hate-to-cause-a-stink-fcc-chairman-declines-call-to-investigate-alleged-swalwell-flatulence.

Chaucer, Geoffrey. *The Canterbury Tales.* New York: Modern Library, 1994.

Chavers, Penny. "Whoopee Cushions and Prank Phone Calls: The Oldest Tricks in the Book." *Curious Historian,* July 31, 2019. https://curioushistorian.com/whoopee-cushions-and-prank-phone-calls-the-oldest-tricks-in-the-book.

Chrisafis, Angelique. "Scotland Yard Recoils from a Foul Wind." *The Guardian,* June 6, 2001. https://www.theguardian.com/uk/2001/jun/07/angeliquechrisafis.

Crick, Robert Alan. *The Big Screen Comedies of Mel Brooks.* Jefferson, NC: McFarland, 2002.

Dawson, Jim. *Blame It on the Dog.* Berkeley: Ten Speed Press, 1999.

Dawson, Jim. *Who Cut the Cheese?* Berkeley: Ten Speed Press, 2006.

Diamond, Jason. "Judd Apatow on Documenting the Legacy (and Fart Jokes) of George Carlin." *Vulture*, May 2022. https://www.vulture.com/2022/05/judd-apatow-george-carlin-documentary-interview.html.

Dicker, Ron. "Stephen Colbert Has a Gas with Doctor's Warning on Farts Spreading Coronavirus." *HuffPost*, April 22, 2020. https://www.huffpost.com/entry/stephen-colbert-farts-coronavirus_n_5ea01b0dc5b6b2e5b83a913a.

Ebert, Roger. "Women Can Get Drunk and Be Crude Too." *Roger Ebert*, May 11, 2011. https://www.rogerebert.com/reviews/bridesmaids-2011.

Farrell, Warren. *The Myth of Male Power.* New York: Berkeley Books, 1993.

Fielding, Henry. *The History of Tom Jones—A Foundling.* New York: Penguin Classics, 2005.

Furz, Peter. *Tailwinds: The Language of Fizzles, Farts and Toots.* London: Michael O'Mara Books, 1998.

Gaiman, Neil, and Kim Newman. *Ghastly Beyond Belief.* New York: Random House Group, 1985.

Garner, Dwight. "Stop the Steal, Giuliani's Flatulence, a Reichstag Moment." *The Irish Times*, July 22, 2021. https://www.irishtimes.com/culture/books/stop-the-steal-giuliani-s-flatulence-a-reichstag-moment-trump-s-apocalyptic-final-year-1.4625864.

Gladwell, Malcom. *David and Goliath: Underdogs, Misfits and the Art of Battling Giants.* New York: Little Brown and Company, 2015.

Glaister, Dan. "Goldberg Dropped from Diet Ads Over Bush Joke." *The Guardian,* July 16, 2004. https://www.theguardian.com/world/2004/jul/16/uselections2004.film.

Gleiberman, Owen. "The Nutty Professor." *Entertainment,* June 28, 1996. https://ew.com/article/1996/06/28/nutty-professor-2/.

Glosswitch. "Why Farting Is a Feminist Issue." *New Statesman,* December 9, 2014. https://www.newstatesman.com/politics/2014/12/why-bodily-functions-are-feminist-issue.

Goldberg, Whoopi. *Book.* New York: Weisbach Books, 1997.

Hemingway, Ernest. *Earnest Hemingway 88 Poems,* edited by Nicholas Gerogiannis. New York: Abe Press, 1979.

Holm, Luke. "An Analysis of 'The Miller's Tale' in Geoffrey Chaucer's *The Canterbury Tales.*" *Owlcation,* July 8, 2022. https://owlcation.com/humanities/An-Analysis-of-The-Millers-Tale-in-Geoffrey-Chaucers-The-Canterbury-Tales.

Irving, David. *The Secret Diaries of Hitler's Doctor.* New York: Macmillan, 1983.

Japiske, Carl, ed. *Fart Proudly: Writings of Benjamin Franklin You Never Read in School.* Columbus, OH: Enthea Press, 1990.

Jennings, Thom. "Comedian Nikki Glaser Not All She Appears." *Niagara Gazette,* October 15, 2014. https://www.niagara-gazette.com/news/night_and_day/comedian-nikki-glaser-not-all-she-appears/article_3cbe0924-18ae-5f5f-835e-67012d99ec67.amp.html.

Keller, Joel. "Eugene Miriman," *AV Club,* March 28, 2012. https://www.avclub.com/eugene-mirman-1798230562.

Klee, Miles. "Bill O'Reilly and Jimmy Kimmel Chat About Hitler's Farts." *Daily Dot,* February 10, 2015. https://www.dailydot.com/upstream/bill-oreilly-kimmel-hitler-farts/.

Krull, Kathleen, and Paul Brewer. *Fartiste.* New York: Simon & Schuster, 2008.

Lasar, Matthew. "Clear Channel to FCC: Wash XM-Sirius' Mouth Out with Soap." *ArsTechnica,* March 25, 2008. https://arstechnica.com/uncategorized/2008/03/clear-channel-to-fcc-wash-xm-sirius-mouth-out-with-soap/.

Lee, Bruce. "Can Farts Transmit COVID-19 Coronavirus? Here Is What Is Being Said." *Forbes,* April 27, 2020. https://www.forbes.com/sites/brucelee/2020/04/27/can-farts-transmit-covid-19-coronavirus-here-is-what-is-being-said/?sh=50137e82310f.

Lezard, Nicholas. "Farewell to the Master of Farting Around." *The Guardian,* April 12, 2007. https://www.theguardian.com/books/booksblog/2007/apr/12/farewelltoamasteroffartin.

Lowry, Brian. "'George Carlin's American Dream' Finds the Right Words to Capture the Comedy Icon." *CNN,* May 20, 2022. https://www.wral.com/george-carlins-american-dream-finds-the-right-words-to-capture-the-comedy-icon/20291431/.

Mandal, Ananya. "Lifting the Lid on Coronavirus Flatulence." *News Medical Life Sciences,* April 22, 2020. https://www.news-medical.net/news/20200422/Lifting-the-lid-on-coronavirus-flatulence.aspx.

McMillan, Dawn. *My Butt Is So Noisy.* Mineola, NY: Dover Publications, 2021.

Mead, Nancy. "Sermon: 'Whatever happened to class.'" *Alamosa News,* May 25, 2018. https://alamosanews.com/article/sermon-whatever-happened-to-class\.

Merrill, John C. *Legacy of Wisdom.* Ames: Iowa State University Press, 1994.

Messner, Michael. *Politics of Masculinities: Men in Movements.* Thousand Oaks, CA: Sage, 1997.

Miller, Daryl H. "Alan Smithee Makes a Name in Hollywood." *Los Angeles Times,* March 5, 2002. https://www.latimes.com/archives/la-xpm-2002-mar-05-et-miller5-story.html.

Miller, Joshua Rhett. "'Panera Karen' Claims Masks Won't Stop COVID-19 Since Pants Don't Contain Farts." *New York Post,* July 22, 2020. https://nypost.com/2020/07/22/panera-karen-masks-dont-stop-covid-19-since-pants-dont-contain-farts/.

Moinzadeh, Atoosah. "Texas Protesters Hold 'Mass Farting' to Counter Pro-Gun Group's Fake Mass Shooting." *Vice,* December 12, 2015. https://www.vice.com/en/article/3kw5jb/texas-protesters-hold-mass-farting-to-counter-pro-gun-groups-fake-mass-shooting.

Molloy, Antonia. "California Killings: Elliot Rodger's parents knew of massacre on radio as they raced to stop their son." *Independent,* May 27, 2014. https://www.independent.co.uk/news/world/americas/california-killings-elliot-rodger-s-parents-heard-about-massacre-on-radio-as-they-raced-to-stop-their-son-9435197.html.

Moore, Tracy. "If You Love Someone, Let Her Fart." *Mel Magazine,* April 7, 2017. https://medium.com/mel-magazine/if-you-love-someone-let-her-fart-616483145e52.

Moss, Candida. "How a Fart Killed 10,000 People." *The Daily Beast,* July 23, 2019. https://www.thedailybeast.com/how-a-fart-killed-10000-people.

Moye, David. "Suspect's Loud Fart Helps Police Sniff Out His Hiding Place." *HuffPost,* July 10, 2019. https://www.huffpost.com/entry/farting-suspect-arrested-liberty-missouri_n_5d2602a6e4b07e698c441405.

Neider, Charles. *The Outrageous Mark Twain.* New York: Doubleday, 1987.

Nohain, Jean, and F. Caradec. *LePetomaine,* Los Angeles: Sherbourne Press, 1967.

Pickett, Calder M. *Voices of the Past: Key Documents in the History of American Journalism.* New York: John Wiley & Sons, 1977.

Pomeroy, Ross. "Women's Farts Smell Worse, and Five More Facts You Need to Know About Flatulence." *RealClearScience,* October 2, 2014. https://www.realclearscience.com/blog/2014/10/6_facts_you_need_to_know_about_farts.html.

Preskar, Peter. "Adolf Hitler Farted Like a Horse." *medium.com,* May 2, 2021. https://medium.com/short-history/adolf-hitler-farting-b7e27477971b.

Reghay, Nayomi. "Meet the Trans Comedian Making Fart Jokes an Act of Resistance." *Rolling Stone,* October 13, 2017. https://www.rollingstone.com/culture/culture-features/patti-harrison-meet-the-trans-comedian-making-fart-jokes-an-act-of-resistance-196357.

Ryskin, Gregory. "Methane-driven Oceanic Eruptions and Mass Extinctions." *GeoScienceWorld,* September 1, 2003. https://pubs.geoscienceworld.org/gsa/geology/article-abstract/31/9/741/29324/Methane-driven-oceanic-eruptions-and-mass.

Salinger, J.D. *The Catcher in the Rye.* New York: Bantam Books, 1978.

Scharhorst, Gary. *The Life of Mark Twain 1891–1910.* Columbia: University of Missouri Press, 2022.

Setoodeh, Raimin. "Sundance: Daniel Radcliffe's Farting Corpse Movie Prompts Walk-Outs." *Variety,* January 22, 2016. https://variety.com/2016/film/news/daniel-radcliffe-farting-corpse-swiss-army-man-1201686756/.

Shakespeare, William. *The Comedy of Errors.* CreateSpace Independent Publishing, 2016.

Stern, Carly. "Thousand Year History of Flatulists." *Daily Mail*, March 8, 2018. https://www.dailymail.co.uk/femail/article-5474797/The-history-flatulists-comedic-fart-performers.html.

Stern, Howard. *Private Parts*. New York: Simon & Schuster, 1993.

Sullivan, Andrew. "A History of Farting." *The Atlantic*, July 18, 2007. https://www.theatlantic.com/daily-dish/archive/2007/07/a-history-of-farting/226692/.

Swift, Jonathan. "The Benefit of Farting Explain'd," *Booktryst*, May 17, 2012. http://www.booktryst.com/2012/05/jonathan-swift-on-women-who-fart-or.html.

Swift, Jonathan. *Poetical Works*. London: Oxford University Press, 1967.

Topaz, Angry. "Was That a Barking Spider?" *Roller Mountain Girls: Denver*, 2020. https://rockymountainrollergirls.com/member-of-the-month-barking-spider/.

Van Munching, Phillip. *Beer Blast*. New York: New York Times Books, 1997.

Vinson, Irmin. "'So the last shall be first …' Alinsky's Farting Negroes." *Counter-Currents*, September 6, 2016. https://counter-currents.com/2016/09/alinskys-farting-negroes/.

Walker, Alexia. "English Literature vs. American Literature." *The Adroit Journal*, May 1, 2019. https://theadroitjournal.org/2019/05/01/english-literature-vs-american-literature/.

Wilstein, Matt. "What Jon Stewart Learned About Fart Jokes from George Carlin." *Daily Beast*, May 19, 2022. https://finance.yahoo.com/news/jon-stewart-learned-comedy-george-013733822.html.

Zinoman, Jason. "The Strategic Mind of Ali Wong." *New York Times*, May 3, 2018. https://www.nytimes.com/2018/05/03/arts/television/ali-wong-netflix-hard-knock-wife.html.

Index

Milton Keynes UK
Ingram Content Group UK Ltd.
UKHW020204231223
434861UK00009B/114